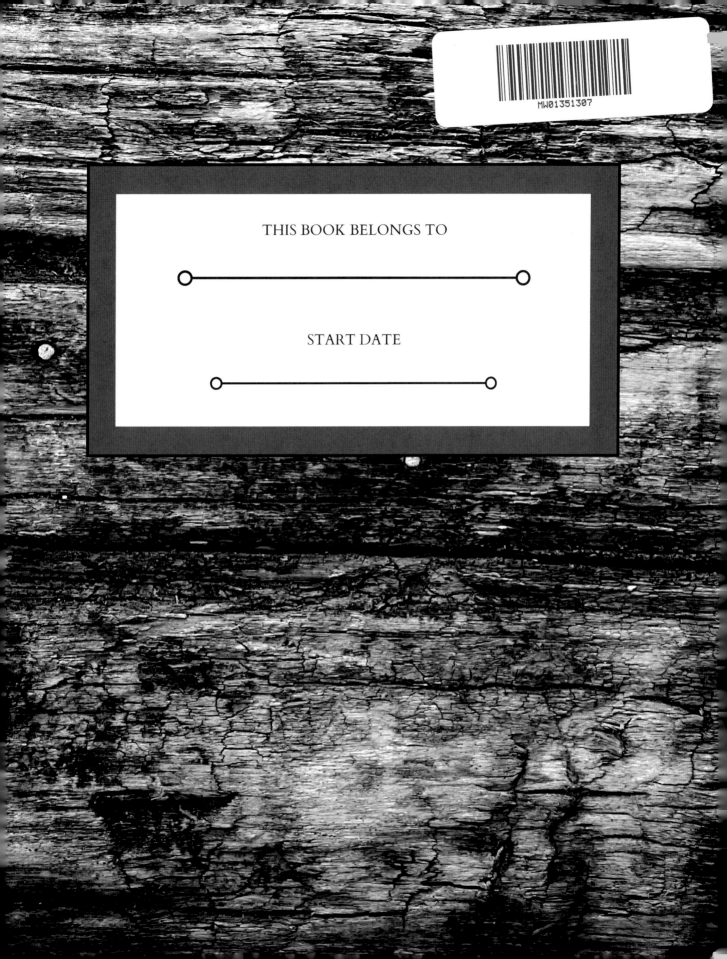

THIS BOOK BELONGS TO

START DATE

EDITORIAL

EDITOR
Donna Christopher

PUBLISHER
Noble International

CREATIVE

GRAPHIC DESIGN
Meagan Hemingson

COVER ART
Rick Schroeppel

PHOTOGRAPHY
Lani Lines p. 114
Adrian Lumi p. 126
Johnny Cohen p. 144
Anthony Intraversato p. 156
Ben White p.184

All images used by permission.

Cancer Peace University

CancerPeaceUniversity.com

BRAVING THE STORM: COMPANION WORKBOOK

© 2021 by Cancer Peace University, LLC

All Rights Reserved

ISBN: 978-0-578-88691-6

No part of this publication may be reproduced, distributed, or transmitted in any formor by any means, including photocopying, recording, or other electronicor mechanical methods, without the prior written permission of Cancer Peace University, LLC, except in the case of brief quotations embodied in critical reviews and certain other noncommercial uses permitted by copyright law.

BRAVING THE STORM
COMPANION WORKBOOK

IN PURSUIT OF A PROFOUND, INTERNAL TRANSFORMATION

This workbook is best used alongside the book, *Braving The Storm: Find Hope During A Cancer Diagnosis.* Chapter by chapter, you will do exercises to help apply the knowledge you are gaining throughout reading the book. The goal is to trigger a profound, internal transformation that will impact your biology.

For added community and conversation, join us in the **Cancer Peace University Facebook Group**!

DISCLAIMER

None of the material in this book is meant to diagnose or treat a disease such as cancer. If you have cancer or suspect you have cancer, schedule an appointment with an oncologist to be treated. The information in this book is not meant to be taken as medical advice or treatment of cancer. If you choose to implement dietary, lifestyle changes and addressing the emotional roots of cancer without consulting your physician or oncologist, which is your constitutional right, you are, in effect, prescribing for yourself. When in doubt of the appropriateness of any protocol, please consult a physician or oncologist. Information in this book and workbook should not be used as a substitute for an oncologist's advice. It is our hope that you do choose a physician or oncologist who realizes the importance of a diet, lifestyle choices and emotional links during a cancer diagnosis. Please be aware that you have the right to make your own health decisions based on any information made available to you through multiple sources including the information from Cancer Peace University. YOU are the driving force in guiding yourself on a path to Abundant Health!

Self-help strategies can be helpful to all people. However, if you have experienced severe trauma and are suffering from PTSD or other conditions related to trauma, this book and workbook are not meant to substitute work with a professional who is trained to help in cases of psychological trauma. Many people will need to pursue professional help to resolve past trauma and PTSD. If at any point while reading the book Braving The Storm and doing the workbook, you are triggered from past trauma that is unresolved, pursue help through a professional, licensed psychiatrist, or counselor trained to help in cases of PTSD and trauma.

Table of Contents

Introduction..................7
Epigenetic Healing

Section 1
Geting Right With Me

Chapter 1 20
A Change of Mind:
The Journey From
Negativity to Positivity
is not as far as you Think

Chapter 2 25
Releasing Regret & Shame:
I am not my Worst Mistake

Chapter 3 31
Freeing Your Mind from
Imprints of Trauma

Chapter 4 46
Embracing Your Eccentricity

Chapter 5 53
Digging Deeper

Section 2
Relationships Reflect Me:
What Do You See?

Chapter 1 64
The Broken Heart

Chapter 2 72
My Soul Deserves Peace

Chapter 3 80
Into Me You See

Chapter 4 84
Come Out of Hiding

Chapter 5 101
The Art of Developing True
Intimacy

Section 3
Unraveling the Imprint of
Trauma

Chapter 1 114
The Dream-Like State of
Surviving Trauma & How to
Move Past Surviving into
Thriving

Chapter 2 118
Mindfulness: Ending the
Phantom Existence

Chapter 3 131
Become a Curious Observer of
Your Internal World & Own Your
Emotional Brain

Chapter 4 144
Reversing the Amnesia of Trauma
to Fully Integrate Your Brain

Chapter 5 156
Healing the Abandoned Heart

Section 4
Wakefulness

Chapter 1 160
Wake up to Spiritual Reality

Chapter 2 164
We all Have an Incurable Disease

Conclusion 186

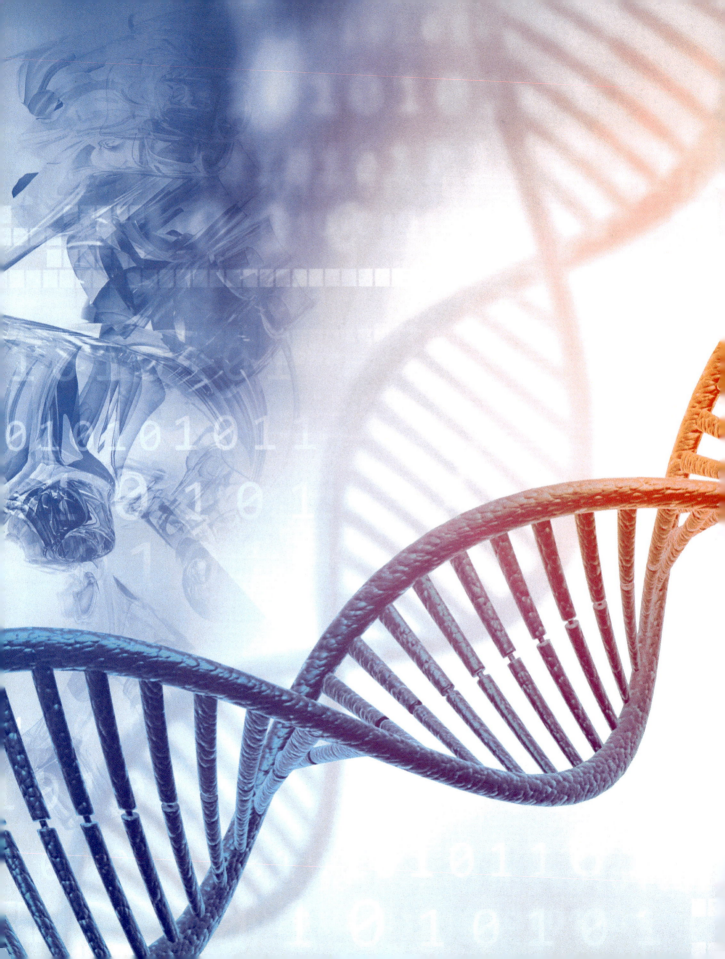

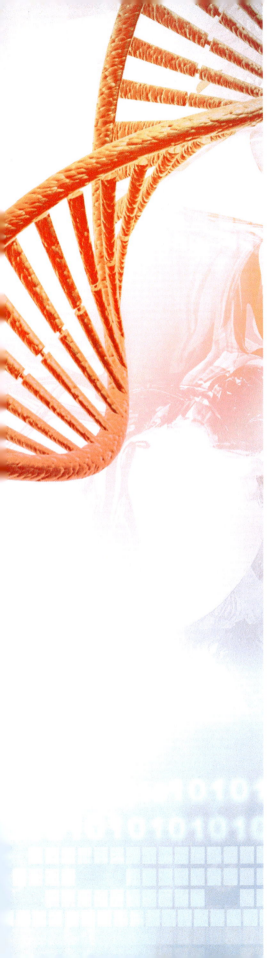

Section 1: Getting Right With Me

Introduction

Epigenetic Healing

Epigenetics Defined:

Epigenetics is the study of how genes interact within the body. Epigenetics explores how our thoughts, beliefs, emotions and lifestyle all serve to stimulate genetic expression or the silencing of genes. This is a fascinating field of study that validates us as whole people with many facets that can either contribute to health or dysfunction and disease. Our goal is to reverse emotional and spiritual rooted stimuli, which have led to physical dysfunction, symptoms or disease.

Concealed Truths

We all carry concealed truths in our subconscious mind that guide our thoughts, emotions and decisions. These truths were created through subjective personal experiences in which we made subconscious decisions on what to believe about the world, others and ourselves. These decisions or conclusions result in our worldview or paradigm in which we interpret the world around us.

Our worldview is developed by 7 years of age, which some live out and express until the day of their death without challenging any beliefs. Many concealed truths are not beneficial to our lives. These maladaptive beliefs create chronic underlying stress in our daily lives, relational interactions and impede our success in life. Maladaptive core beliefs can also create dysfunction in our physical body.

Our goal is to gain access to these concealed truths or maladaptive core beliefs to create new meaning in our lives. Further, we desire to understand critical events from our past so that we can shift our emotional, psychological and spiritual paradigms in a direction that is positive and life-giving to our body, soul and spirit.

First, let's look at a diagram of our soul so that we can understand the components of our soul.

MIND
Thoughts, beliefs, subconscious beliefs, imagination and basic assumptions

WILL
Action, behavior, internal and external decisions & inner vows

SOUL

EMOTIONS
Hot & cold emotions: anger, rage, sadness, depression, hopelessness, etc; present emotional reality and past emotional reality

We all have encountered experiences and interactions with family members, friends and coworkers that have left a negative impression on our souls. Our interpretation of these events, how we process and evaluate ourselves in relation to others, will determine our emotional health moving forward. Many times, it is the events in our past that imprinted trauma upon our soul, which needs to be re-evaluated with new information and fresh perspective. In this manner, we can resolve concealed truths that impinge upon our ability to move forward in the direction of emotional and physical wholeness.

The subconscious mind stores our core belief system or worldview in the form of memories. The process of building our worldview begins in the womb and continues until we are 7 years of age. Thus, the first 7 years of our lives are critical to the rest of our lives! Many of us have negative experiences and even trauma that occurred during this crucial time frame. The conclusions that we made during negative experiences in childhood frame our worldview.

For example, when I was 7 years old, I had a negative experience with a teacher who disciplined me very harshly in front of my entire classroom. She demanded that I go to the classroom next door, tell the teacher that I was in trouble and ask her to give me a desk to sit in while I wrote "I will not talk in class" 50 times.

Because I was embarrassed and humiliated in such a dramatic fashion, I came to the conclusion that I was rejected.

This caused me to become more introverted and calculating in how I interacted with others instead of being spontaneous and free in my expression.

Our goal in the exercises of this workbook is to discover pivotal moments in your childhood and life that defined your perception of reality in a negative light. Once you have accessed these memories, we will work to reinterpret these experiences in a way to shift your subconscious belief system or worldview.

IDENTITY

The spiritual side of our identity is an important component to the health and wholeness of our identity as an individual. Here is the breakdown of the components to your identity.

PHYSICAL

Height, weight, health, how you feel, how you take care of your body and express your physical self in the world

SOUL

MIND:
Your subconscious and conscious beliefs, thought patterns and knowledge through personal and professional growth shape your unique mind. Imagination: Whom do you imagine yourself to be in the future? What is the image you have in your mind of who you are? How was this image formed?

WILL:
Your daily decisions develop into habits that express your deepest beliefs, assumptions and vision of your life and how you can best contribute to the world.

PERSONALITY:
What makes you unique? What are your unique strengths? Your unique attributes include your gifts, what you value, how you express your emotions, thoughts and beliefs. Personality can also include your hobbies, passions and pursuits along with whether you internally or externally process your thoughts and emotions. Are you an introvert or an extrovert?

SPIRIT:
What do you believe about God, the spiritual world and what happens after you die? What is your purpose and meaning in life?
How do you develop your unique contribution to the world around you? How do you express and grow in your spiritual beliefs and practices? How do you connect with God and the spiritual world? The spiritual side of a person includes listening and becoming congruent with our conscience about individual and personal transactions.

EMOTIONS:
What do you feel and how deeply do you feel it? What moves you to compassion and love? What soul wounds do you carry from your past and how does it impact your relationships? How aware are you of your emotions and how do you express them? Have you developed your emotional intelligence through self-awareness? How deeply are you able to connect with yourself and others emotionally?

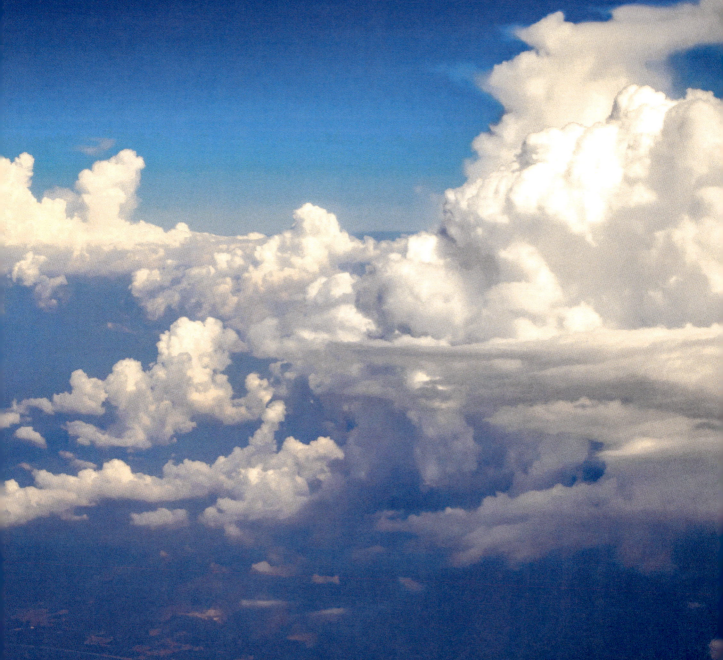

"We are not human beings having a spiritual experience. We are spiritual beings having a human experience."
~Teilhard de Chardin

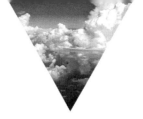

Three Requirements for Participants

1. A desire to change at least one specific feeling or behavior that you no longer want in your life.

2. A commitment to the truth no matter how strange.

3. A willingness to experiment, which may require a sense of humor :)

Benefits of Epigentic Healing

1. A change in unwanted feelings and behaviors.

2. More conscious choice in stuck areas of your life.

3 Greater self-respect - much greater!

4. Transformation to your thoughts, emotions, spirit and physical health!

5. Ultimately, you will become a more centered and mature person by confronting concealed truths and allowing your worldview to shift towards a positive direction.

LET'S GET STARTED!
FIRST OF ALL:

Relax

You probably won't discover what you need to discover while under stress. We have more than one attempt at this and I am here to help you.

First impressions are often the most valuable in this healing process, even if they seem totally weird. When you read the questions that I am asking, I would like you to reply with the **very first** thought that comes to mind without editing or judging the thought.

Open-mindedness: When was the last time you felt open-minded?

Picture yourself in the stage of your life that you were the most open-minded.

What did you look like? What did it feel like to be in your body and mind? If it has been a while, I want you to imagine that you are magically more open-minded than you have ever been.

Did you know that open-minded people have a stronger sense of self?

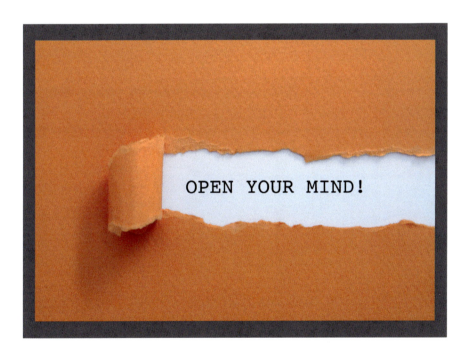

It is healthy and mature to be open-minded. Are you feeling open-minded now? If you aren't, then you might want to wait to do epigenetic healing until you are open-minded and ready to heal.

Why is open-mindedness so important?

Open-mindedness allows us to bypass psychological defense mechanisms in our mind. Physical defense mechanisms (like fortresses) are designed to resist pain (like being shot or stabbed). Psychological defense mechanisms are intended to resist emotional pain. When we resist or deny conscious awareness of emotional pain, we are prevented from ever doing anything about it. And this only creates more pain that you feel compelled to resist. It becomes a vicious cycle.

*Is it time for you to get out of this viscious cycle
of suppressing emotional pain?*

Then decide now to open your
mind to the truth–
truth you may have never considered
or truth that you have always "sort of"
known but have never really acknowledged.
Ok?

Tell the truth. You can handle it.

Now, I hope you understand more about your soul, spirit and epigenetic healing. We can make changes and new decisions with new information on how our emotions are connected to past events, traumas and beliefs that were set in motion based upon our perceptions of childhood experiences.

Our goal in the coming pages of this workbook is to help you connect with your emotions, move through your emotions to connect with your beliefs, make the subconscious conscious and to shift the paradigm of your soul to a new place of awareness and wholeness.

To do that, you will need to set aside the defense mechanisms that keep you in denial. This is why open-mindedness is so important. Open-mindedness is the opposite of denial and resistance.

Now, answer the following questions with the most **open-minded & honest** answers that you can and discover what you need to know in order to experience a profound, internal transformation!

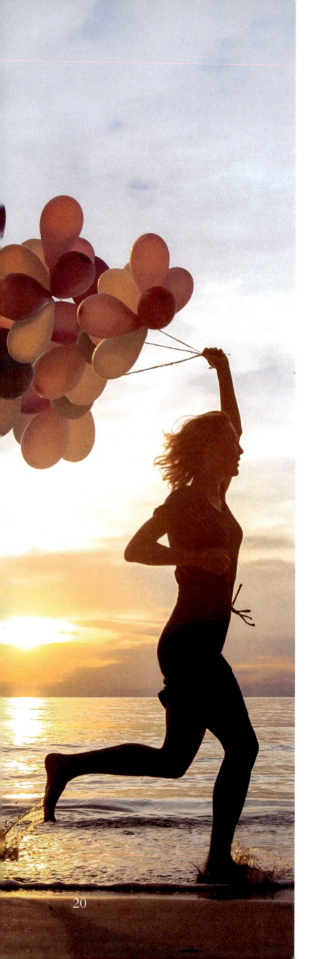

Section 1: Getting Right With Me

Chapter 1

A Change of Mind

The Journey From Negativity to Positivity is not as far as you Think

What is the biggest thing that impacted you from this chapter and why?

Did you know it was possible to move from a pessimistic person to an optimistic person? Do you want to become more positive? Explain.

What are some negative thoughts that you notice in your mind on a regular basis?

How do you feel when you think these thoughts?

Now, close your eyes and follow the feeling to a memory, what memory do you have from your past where you felt the same way that you are feeling now?

How did that experience impact your life?

Do you have a diagnosed disease currently or in the past?

What were the circumstances of your life when the diagnosis occurred?

> [*Be open and think about every possibility: the death of a loved one, moving to another house or location, breaking up with a boyfriend or going through a divorce, etc. Remember that an emotional trauma is subject to interpretation. Small, insignificant things can be emotionally traumatic to a child.*]

Write down the first thing that comes to mind when you think of a potential emotional root to your cancer diagnosis:

If you cannot find words to describe why you have cancer, try to draw a picture that shows why you have cancer. After you draw the picture, write what you see.

....

....

What are some of the emotions that you experience on a daily or weekly basis that are troublesome to you (for example, extreme anger, frustration, despair, depression, sadness, hopelessness, fear…)?

If you struggle to identify your emotions, try the following exercise. Draw a picture of how you feel right now in your life. After you draw the picture, write what you see and how you feel:

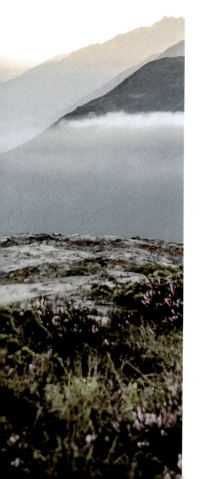

Any major or minor trauma that happened in your childhood or adult life that could be unresolved?

If you are unsure or cannot connect with this exercise, try to draw a picture of an unresolved event from childhood. After you draw the picture, try to write down what you see.

What needs to change in your life in order for you to heal?

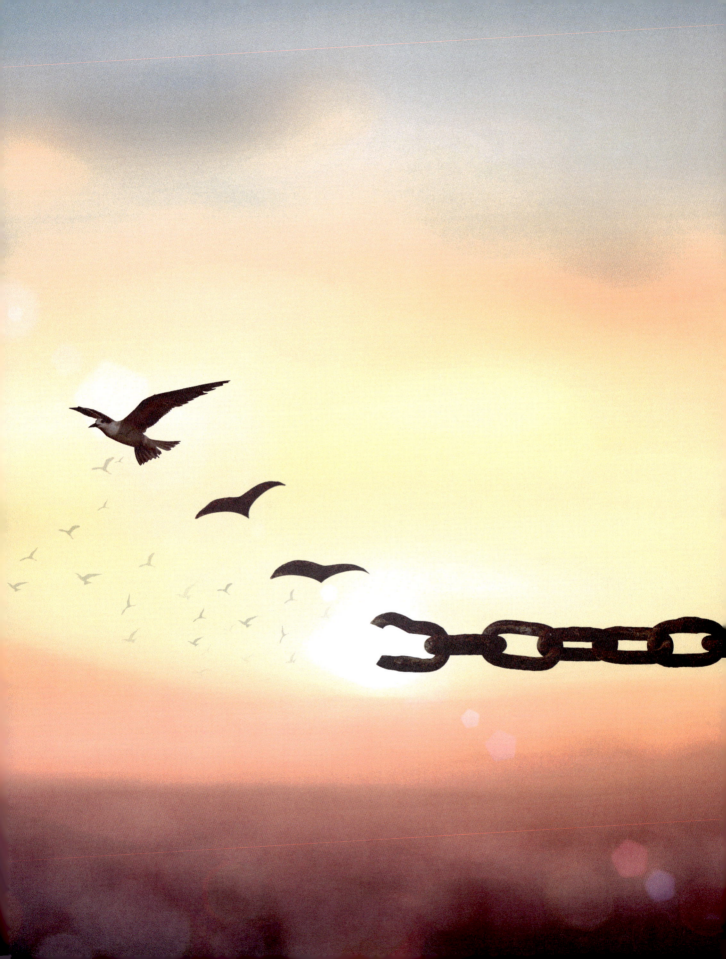

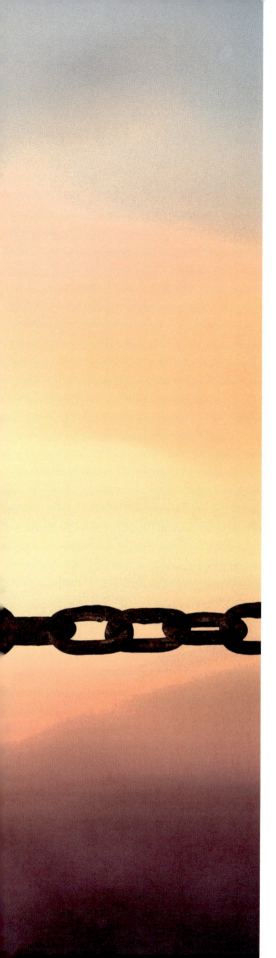

Section 1: Getting Right With Me

Chapter 2

Releasing Regret & Shame

I Am Not My Worst Mistake

Exercise on Regrets, Mistakes, Transgressions & New Starts:

Do you have any regrets?

What do you regret doing or not doing in your life?

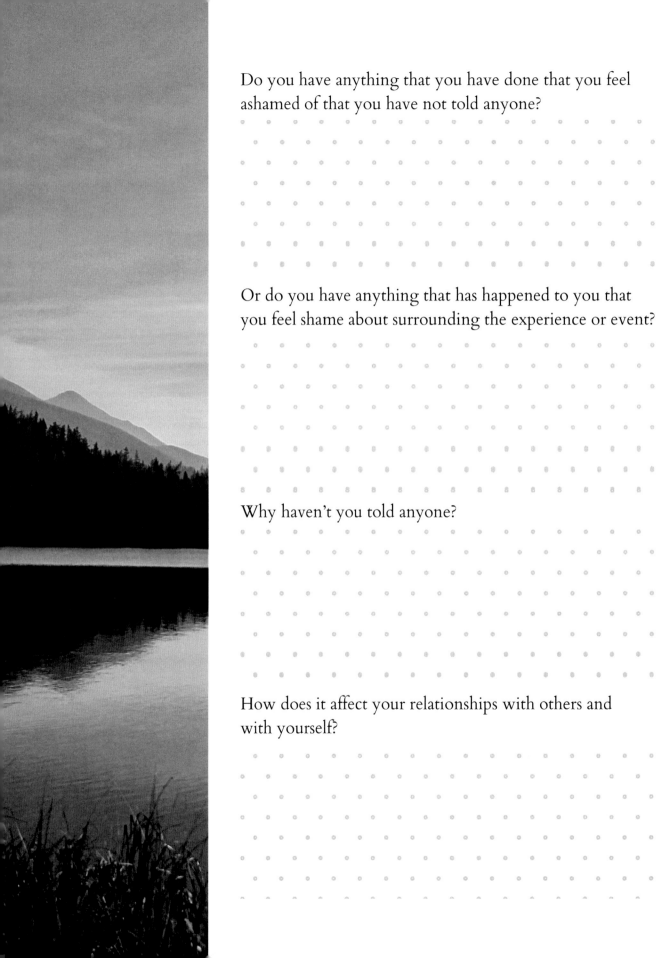

Do you have anything that you have done that you feel ashamed of that you have not told anyone?

Or do you have anything that has happened to you that you feel shame about surrounding the experience or event?

Why haven't you told anyone?

How does it affect your relationships with others and with yourself?

Find one person whom you trust and share your regrets with them in a letter or in person and ask them to forgive you for your transgressions. Receive their love, understanding and forgiveness, as if it was the person whom you hurt.

> Also, if you had a traumatic experience as a child or as an adult, find someone whom you can trust to share this trauma with to find freedom from the weight of shame *(A word of caution: Be careful whom you pick; find a trustworthy person who can show empathy and love without any judgment. Make sure that you arrange a time to share with the person to allow ample time for the person to listen and show empathy in order to ensure that this experience is healing and doesn't re-traumatize you).*

Write what happened here:

If you don't feel ready to do the exercise above or you don't have someone whom you trust with deep pain or shame, continue to write every day for 15-20 minutes about what happened to you. Each day that you write, express what happened, how you felt, how it impacted you in the past and how it impacts your life now. Try to write one good thing that came out of that experience (if you can find something good).

What happened (regret or trauma)?

How did you feel?

How did it impact your life at the time?

How does it impact your life now?

EXTRA JOURNALING & DRAWING SPACE

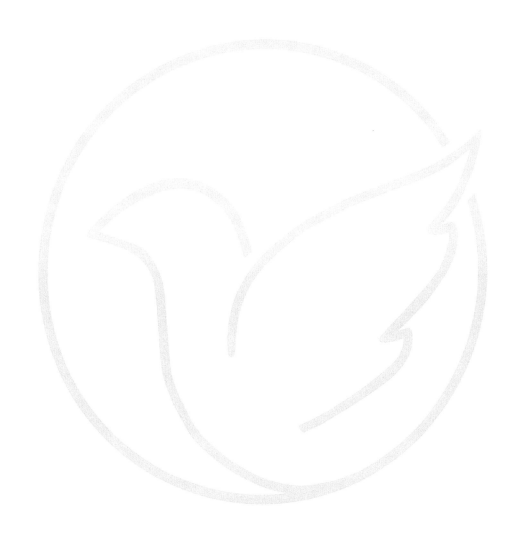

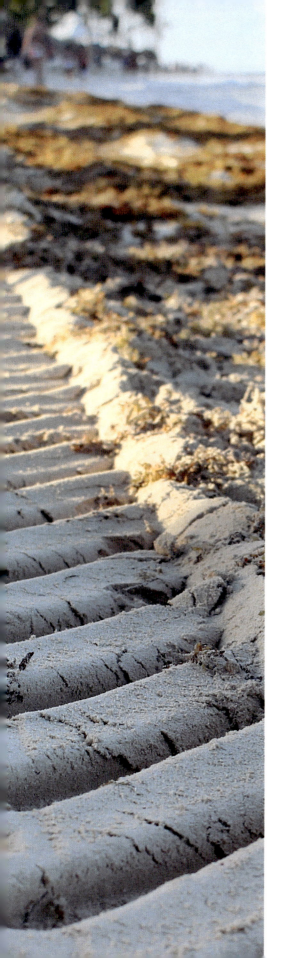

Section 1: Getting Right With Me

Chapter 3

Freeing Your Mind From Imprints of Trauma

Exercise for healing from childhood trauma:

Create a timeline of emotional and relational trauma. Keep in mind that trauma is based upon our perception. A seemingly small, insignificant moment in your life can impact you in a major way.

When you write down your timeline of trauma consider and include moments of pain, rejection, fear, negative experiences and those moments where you have vivid memories that hold strong emotions.

As an adult, I didn't have a lot of childhood memories, but the memories that kept surfacing for me were defining moments. These defining moments caused me to change the way I viewed the world, others and even led me to adjust my personality. Also, the memories that surfaced were vivid with strong emotions that felt alive and still active.

I will share my "Timeline of Trauma" to help you see what this process can look like:

Megan's Timeline of Trauma

1. My 2nd grade teacher disciplined me by sending me to the next-door classroom to write, "I will not talk in class" 50 times. I was embarrassed and felt very rejected. This was a defining moment in a negative light because I changed my personality after this to become more introverted, calculated and less spontaneous.

2. I broke my arm. My brother and I were racing up the ladder to the slide at the same time and I fell off the side of the ladder. My mom didn't think that I was seriously injured because we had been bothering her all day with little fights. Thus, my brother had to walk me up to the house to show my mom that I was seriously injured.

3. We moved to a new house and I started to go to a new school in 3rd grade. I was scared and I didn't know anyone at the new school.

4. My dad started working a lot more when he bought my grandpa's business. I felt his energy shift from home to work. I was "Daddy's Girl" and I missed my dad's attention and affection. I made a decision to strive and work really hard to excel in order to get my dad's attention and affection again.

5. I cried about my body image in elementary school to my mom. I felt hurt when she gave me advice to stop eating ice cream. I think that I just wanted a hug and to be told that I was beautiful no matter what. As a result, I decided not to cry in front of women anymore. For 11 years, I didn't cry in front of women until I redesigned the memory as an adult.

6. My best friend moved to Europe.

7. I was in a lot of competitions for figure skating, but I never won. After every competition, I always cried because I never felt good enough or perfect enough.

8. In 8th grade, I felt rejected by my peers and felt conflicted every day at lunch concerning who I should sit next to. I was very self-conscious and never felt good enough.

9. I was caught shoplifting at Target in high school, lost my dad's trust and felt a lot of shame and regret regarding that decision.

10. I moved to Nashville, TN when I was 18 and started college at Vanderbilt University. I started experiencing panic attacks every night.

11. I didn't get into any sorority during the college rush process and I felt like the entire school rejected me.

Hopefully, my timeline of trauma helps you to realize that the small moments in life can be defining moments. You may have experienced a pretty normal childhood with some negative experiences as I had. Or you may have had an abusive, tragic childhood that left you very broken as a result. Either way, we all have had at least a few negative experiences to resolve from childhood.

My Timeline of Trauma

1.

2.

3.

4.

5.

6.

7.

8.

9.

10.

After you write your timeline of trauma, here are some questions to ask yourself:

What triggers you to go into a mode of hurt, pain, anger or trauma? Personally, I was sensitive to rejection and had to address times in my past where I felt rejected in order to move out of the self-perception that "I am rejected."

Now, we are going to work on redesigning memories in your "Timeline of Trauma." Some people find it fairly easy to do the memories on their own. Others struggle to make progress and need someone trained in memory work to help them. Test your memories and see how well you are able to engage in redesigning memories on your own.

NOTES

Instructions for Redesigning Your Memories:

Start with your first memory on your "Timeline of Trauma." Sit in a relaxed environment, with a journal and meditative music.

As you sit, take a deep breath, open your heart and allow yourself to walk through the memory. **Close your eyes while you focus on the memory, pen in hand.** Notice every emotion and twist and turn in the memory.

Since most people will have many memories, we have written the instructions in the workbook to follow memory by memory. Use your own journal or notebook to answer each question and exercise in redesigning your memories.

Please repeat these instructions to redesign each memory in your timeline.

1. Write down what you notice about the memory as you walk through it.

2. How do you feel in the memory and why?

3. What are the top 3 predominant emotions in the memory?

4. Are there other people in the memory with you?
   How do you feel about the person in the memory when the memory starts?
   How do you feel about the person at the end of the memory?

5. What are your thoughts in the memory?

6. What did you conclude about yourself or life at the end of the memory? (i.e. I am rejected, I am abandoned, I cannot trust anyone ever again, I hate myself, I hate God, etc.)

7. Did you make any decisions in the memory to protect yourself from being hurt again? (i.e. I will never cry in front of anyone again, I will never share my emotions again, I will never trust again)

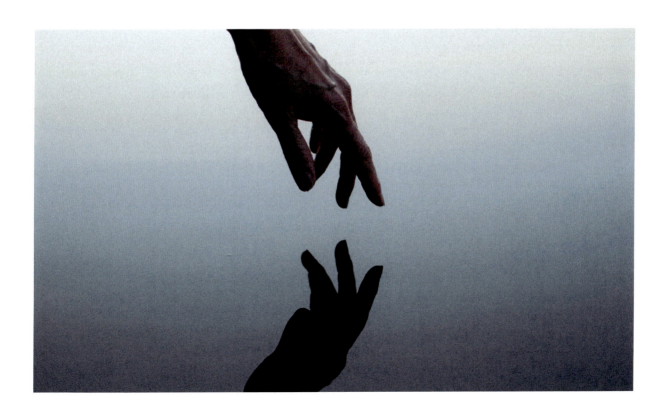

Now that you have the detailed imprint of the memory, go through it slowly to redesign the memory as we guide you.

8. Take some time to forgive.

    Remember that forgiveness is a choice that we make based upon a principle.

    Most of the time, people don't deserve our forgiveness. However, most of us have at least one decision from our lives that we don't deserve forgiveness for either.

    Most of the time, we don't feel like forgiving. Many times, after we forgive, our feelings change towards the person and we feel more compassion. We don't have to enter into a relationship with everyone we forgive, if we are not safe or if the relationship is abusive. **Some relationships are toxic and should not be rebuilt.**

9. Say out loud, **"Today, I choose to forgive you, _____, not because you apologized or because you deserve it, but because my soul needs peace. I forgive you, _____ for _____ and I release any and all offense that I took in this memory.**

10. Once you have forgiven each person including yourself and perhaps God, revisit the memory again. Does the memory feel any different or does it feel the same?

Do you feel less anger and resentment or is it still lingering?

If you are struggling to forgive, you can try these exercises to access forgiveness: Ask God to help you forgive. Say out loud, **"God, can you help me to forgive, _____."** After you ask for help, wait and see what you feel, notice or sense.

Do you see anything in your mind, hear anything or do you feel any different?

"Today I decided to forgive you. Not because you apologized, or because you acknowledged the pain that you caused me, but because my soul deserves peace." — Najwa Zebian

Imagine the person you need to forgive in a very scary, vulnerable situation. The best scenario is to imagine something that you know they have experienced in life or in which they are currently experiencing. Notice how they look, how they feel and how you feel.

Do you notice any feelings of compassion towards them now? If not, keep trying. Write down what you notice in this exercise.

If you feel ready to forgive after asking God for help and after imagining the person in a difficult situation, try to forgive again. Say out loud, **"I choose to forgive, _____, for _____ and I release all offense that I took in this memory towards them and towards God."**

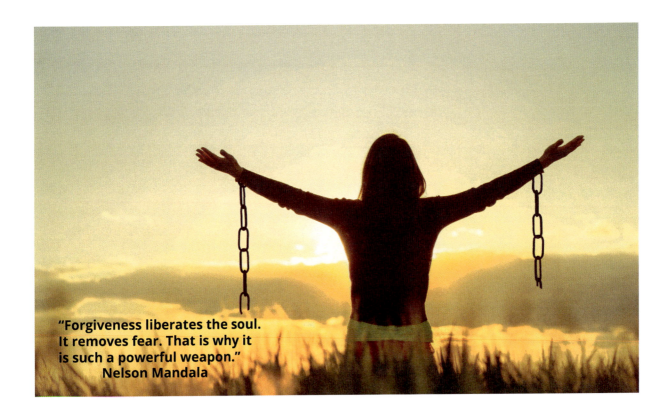

"Forgiveness liberates the soul. It removes fear. That is why it is such a powerful weapon."
Nelson Mandala

11. Check the memory again. How does it feel now?

    You may need to forgive many times, until it is all gone.

12. Notice what emotions are still lingering in the memory.
    Do you feel shame, rejection, sadness, betrayal or abandonment?

    What are the deepest emotions that you can pinpoint in this memory?

    There may be other things to address in the memory. You may need to release certain emotions from yourself like shame, self-hatred, self-bitterness, pain, trauma or sadness and you can do this by saying:
    "I release myself from the shame of this memory, the self-hatred that I embraced, the pain, the sadness and the trauma that have lingered in my life. I choose to be free."

13. Further, examine the memory for decisions, inner vows or ways in which you changed your personality after this experience. Many times, we conclude something about life or make a decision to change ourselves to avoid emotional pain again.

    Have you made any inner decisions that you need to address?

Memories are malleable to the point where we can change decisions that we made to protect ourselves from emotional pain. To make a new decision, say the following out loud:

"I no longer want to protect and hide myself out of pain, rejection, trauma or betrayal. I do not want this past experience to color my life in a negative way any longer.

I choose to make a new decision in this memory to feel emotions, to connect with others and to express myself in a healthy manner. More specifically, I choose to break the inner decision that I made to _____(i.e. stop crying in front of men or women, to shut down my emotions, hate myself, hurt myself, not trust again, etc...).

I make a new decision to _____(i.e. cry in front of people, trust again, love myself, not hurt myself, etc...)."

> After breaking any inner vows, how does the memory feel now?
>
> Notice any changes in your personality or expression of emotions after this exercise.

14. If you rejected yourself or started to hate yourself after this experience, close your eyes and picture yourself as an adult entering into the memory to say, **"I'm sorry that you had this horrible experience. You felt alone, hurt, abandoned and misunderstood. As a result, you started to reject and hate yourself. I love you and I don't hate you. I don't reject you."** Now, give your younger self a hug in the memory.

    After the hug, say this out loud, **"Although I went through this horrible experience, I no longer choose to reject or hate myself. Instead, I choose to love myself and show myself the kindness that I needed at the time of this memory and that I still need."**

    How does the memory feel after this exercise?

15. If you still have lingering emotions, or if you felt like a victim and never expressed certain emotions to the person who hurt you, now is your chance to do this. Go into the memory and address the person who hurt you. Say what you were unable to say or express emotionally at the time of the memory. Say it out loud.

16. Now is the part of the memory work where we invite God into the memory. Hold the memory in your mind and say the following out loud, **"I invite God to come into this memory to restore me."**
You can also ask God a question, **"God, what do you see or how do you feel about me in this memory?"**

Now, wait for God to come into the memory or show you something. Wait for a response like you would if you asked a friend a question. Whatever you see, feel, sense or hear, write it down.

What did you notice after you invited God into the memory?

After you receive something, check the memory again. How does the memory feel now?

After you complete 1 memory and feel like it is resolved, you can work on the next one.
You probably need to focus on one memory at a time.
You may need to do some memories more than once if they hold a lot of pain. You also may need to enlist the help of someone trained in memory work.

EXTRA JOURNALING & DRAWING SPACE

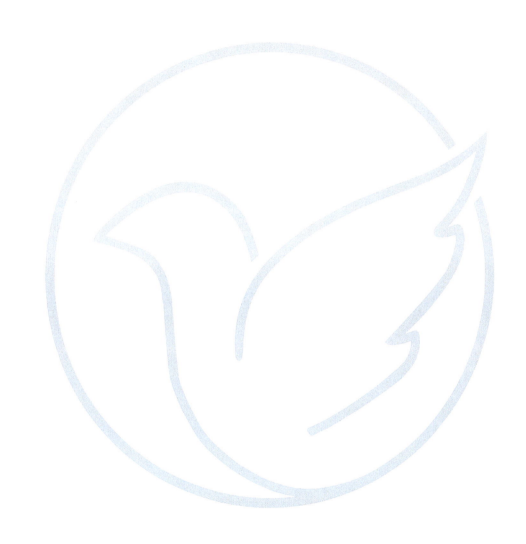

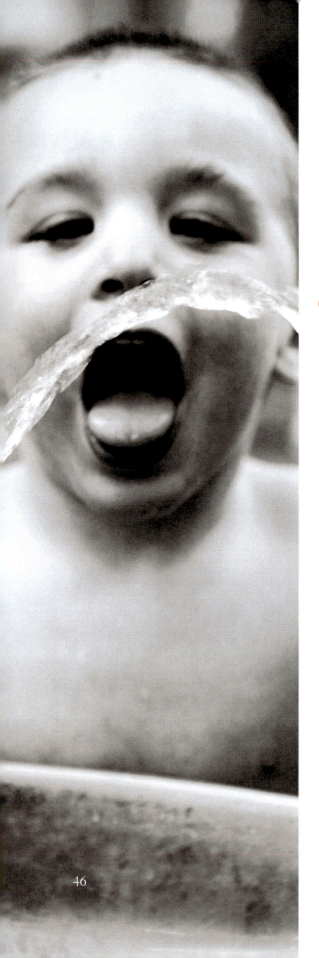

Section 1: Getting Right With Me

Chapter 4

Embracing Your Eccentricity

Let's do an exercise to work on any potential personality traits that you have that may be correlated with a cancer diagnosis. Here are the personality traits found to be common with "The Type C Personality."

Simply put a check mark by the traits that you recognize in yourself:

- ____ Cooperative
- ____ Passive
- ____ Accepting
- ____ Lacking Assertiveness
- ____ Emotional repression
- ____ Pushing down emotions
- ____ Avoiding conflict
- ____ Wanting to be liked

_____ Denial

_____ Repression of anger

_____ Restricted emotions

_____ Aggressive emotions related to your own needs being restricted

_____ Poor ability to cope with stress

_____ Responsible, caring

_____ Tendency to take on the burdens of others

_____ A deep desire to make others happy (people-pleaser)

_____ Harboring suppressed toxic emotions

_____ Inability to express and resolve deep emotional conflicts or unaware of their presence

_____ History of lack of closeness with one or both parents, lack of closeness with spouse

_____ Coping style with stress: denial, avoidance & suppression

Take some time to assess your own personality and internal processing habits as it relates to "The Type C Personality."

What traits do you exhibit in your own life and why?

How did you develop these personality traits?

Granted, some of these traits aren't negative or unhealthy by themselves. However, taken to the extreme, these traits can cause an imbalance that can lead to higher stress levels than a person can cope with (*If you are unsure as to how to answer these questions and of which character traits from "The Type C Personality" that you possess, ask those closest to you to give their assessment. Sometimes, we have blind spots and people close to us have insight in this area*).
What feedback did you receive from your friends and family members?

Are you known as the caretaker of your family?

Do you have the proper time to care for your own needs emotionally, physically and spiritually?

Do you alter how you share and express yourself to make yourself more "socially acceptable" or to avoid any conflict? Explain.

Pick 1 character trait every 2 weeks to 1 month to actively change your way of engaging in this area. For example, if you tend to repress emotions, work on learning to identify your feelings and share them with people close to you.

This may be a messy, difficult process, but it will be worth it. Tell those who are close to you that you are doing an experiment to learn how to express emotions, to become more proactive or to stop taking on the role of the caretaker so that they are prepared for the changes.

> Facing a near death experience can end up being a doorway to a new life. When people face a cancer diagnosis, they can find courage and even permission to stop living the way that everyone expects them to live and to do what is in their heart.
>
> Dr. Hamer coined the phrase "psycho-emotional isolation" to describe the phenomenon of his cancer patients inability to emotionally connect. He found cancer patients to not only be isolated from others emotionally, but also to be isolated from themselves, not understanding or expressing their deepest emotions.

Do you find yourself in a state of psycho-emotional isolation?

Why?

How did you develop this state of isolation?

Let's look at your life as a novel in which you are the author. The publisher calls you one day and says that they are ready to bring out the second edition. What are the things that you want to change in your novel for the second edition of your book? How would you design a way of life for you that you will enjoy for a long period of time?

Build your second edition novel here. What is the plot of the story and the themes? What would your best life look like?

[

]

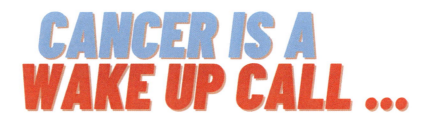

...to take back our lives and to make changes in every area of our lives! It is important to work on both the internal and external aspects of our lives. If we recover the hope that we can live a meaningful and zestful life, our immune system may regain the resources and energy to fight for our life saying, "This individual is worth fighting for."

Many times, people who go through spontaneous remission from cancer find themselves able to surrender to a new way of experiencing themselves with a major shift in their identity.

//

Describe a time in your life that you had the most zest and enthusiasm for life. What was a part of your life that made it so joyful to be alive? How can you recreate this joy?

What is right with you? What are your unique ways of being, relating, creating that are your natural ways of expressing yourself? What is your unique song to sing?

What is your purpose? What do you derive meaning from? What are the puzzle pieces of your identity?

When do you feel the most alive? When and where do you have periods where you lose track of time because you are so engrossed by what you are doing?

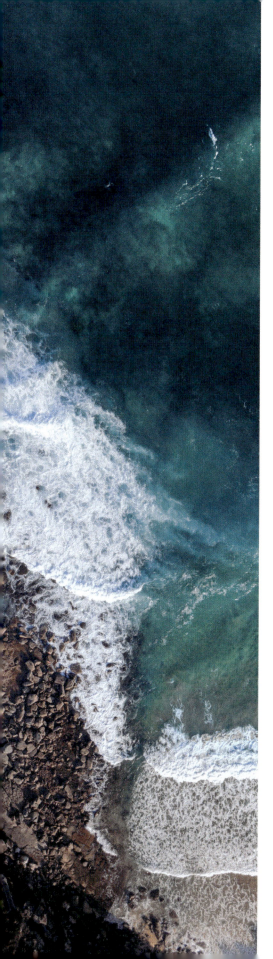

Section 1: Getting Right With Me

Chapter 5

Digging Deeper

Do you have a loved one or spouse that continually tells you that they want to emotionally connect with you, but you don't know what that means?

Do you find yourself figuring out how you feel about a conversation with a loved one days after the conversation instead of in the moment or right after the conversation?

Do you experience intense road rage or other extreme emotions in moments that seem completely inappropriate?

Are you easily able to pinpoint how you feel when you notice bodily sensations or are you often confused about how you feel?

Excerpt from Braving The Storm:

"When trauma victims write about their experiences, physiological changes occur in their bodies including increased blood flow and a boost to the immune system."

DUMPING EXERCISE

A helpful approach to journaling is "free association journaling." This simply means to write down all of your thoughts as they come without judging, editing or blocking them. *Just dump your thoughts in the space below.*

Follow your thoughts to what you notice in your body. Are you noticing anything in your body like pain in a certain area, an increase to your heart rate, an upset stomach, trouble breathing or a desire to cry? If you are, allow yourself to identify the emotion and release it.

Soon, you will learn to identify anxiety with an increased heart rate and racing thoughts. Or fear as an inability to breathe and an upset stomach.

Simply notice what is occurring in your body as you write and write down how your body feels. Ask yourself questions like, my heart is racing and I feel an upset stomach, how do I feel?

                                                                      Why do I feel this way?

At some point in this process, you may feel like crying or screaming. Allow yourself to express your emotions as they come.

The goal of this type of journaling is to connect your thoughts to your emotions and to open yourself up to connect with your subconscious mind, which contains your memories. Your memories hold the keys to understanding your belief system and to finding maladaptive core beliefs that need to shift.

NOTES

You may gain insight into why you feel the way that you feel. After you express an emotion, just listen or watch your mind space for added insight. You may see an image or a memory flash before your mind. Write down the image or memory.

Have you remembered this before?

Do you need to redesign this memory? Follow the steps of redesigning memories in **Chapter 3: Freeing Your Mind From Imprints Of Trauma.**

Exercise: Spend 10-30 minutes per day with free association journaling. Pause as you notice any emotions connected to your thought patterns. Allow expression for that emotion at the moment it appears in your body. Write down any image or memory that comes to your mind.

Exercise: Meditation is a powerful way to connect your conscious mind to your subconscious mind. Once we connect to the subconscious mind, we can gain access to maladaptive core beliefs stored in past memories.

> Your subconscious mind knows exactly what is blocking you from healing and can give your conscious mind the appropriate information at the right time.

In the beginning, it is best to meditate after you have spent time journaling. This way, your mind is less easily distracted with jumbled thoughts.

Pick a phrase to use in meditation. Start with 10-20 minutes per day in meditation. Here are some phrases to pick from:

"God is love."

"He carries our sorrows."

"He Who heals all your diseases."

"I cried out to You and You healed me."

"Who redeems your life from destruction."

"He heals the brokenhearted and binds up their wounds."

"Heal me and I will be healed, save me and I will be saved."

"I will restore health to you."

"To God belongs escape from death."

"Faith is taking the first step even when you don't see the whole staircase."

"Shared joy is a double joy; shared sorrow is half a sorrow."

"Life can only be understood backward, but it must be lived forward."

"People need loving the most when they deserve it the least."

"God speaks in the silence of the heart. Listening is the beginning of prayer."

"The fear of death follows from the fear of life. A man who lives fully is prepared to die at any time."

"Loneliness is the most terrible poverty."

Sit in a comfortable chair, with meditative music, focusing on a phrase that relaxes the body, calms your mind and instructs your subconscious.

When you meditate, take the phrase and rearrange it in your mind. For example, let's work with the following phrase:

God is love.

You could internally think: *God is love. God defines love. God represents love. God is full of love. God loves. God loves me. What is love? God is love. God fills me with love.*

Next, start asking questions and wait for the answer. *Who is God? What is love? How do I receive love?*

//

A client of mine described the first time that she meditated using the phrase, "God is love." She focused on that phrase for 30-minutes, changing it in her mind and receiving the spiritual impact. She was shocked when she felt waves of God's love hitting her body, mind and heart. She felt a calming, beautiful spiritual presence with her as she focused on that phrase. She received the spiritual impact of her meditation. This is the goal of meditation, to receive the spiritual reality of the phrase in order to find spiritual connection.

At the end of the meditation, it is good to pause and listen to any spiritual feedback that comes to you. You might hear a phrase, see an image or feel a sense of peace come over you.

Take the phrase that you were meditating upon and think about it during the day when you have blank space, when you are driving the car or in line at the grocery store, etc. You can use this strategy to shift your consciousness to peace so that you can develop spiritual connection throughout your day.

Next, let's develop your visualization strategy. People who dive deep into healing tend to spend time visualizing their body healing. After meditation, ask for a healing image to focus on. Draw a picture of your healing visualization strategy:

Every day, spend 5 minutes visualizing your healing using this image at the end of your journaling & meditation time.

Finally, let's explore the concepts discovered in The Cunningham Study to examine how open you are to dive deep into emotional healing. For a review of The Cunningham Study, see pages 77-78 in *Braving The Storm:*

1. Do you have low self-esteem or high self-esteem?

    Were you belittled or spoken about negatively during childhood by your caregivers?

    How can you develop higher self-esteem?

2. Are you open to challenging your worldview and changing your belief system to something more life-giving? Why or why not?

3. Do you believe that self-help strategies, self-awareness, journaling, meditation and growing in spiritual connection can assist during a healing process? Why or why not?

4. Do you believe that there is a spiritual realm? Do you believe in life after death? Why or why not?

Are you open to growing spiritually? Why or why not?

5. Do you have a strong will to live? What are you living for?

6. Are you searching for a deeper meaning in your life?

7. What do you believe you are supposed to accomplish on earth?

If you answered the following: *Yes, I have a strong will to live. Yes, I am open to challenging my worldview. Yes, I believe that self-help strategies will help me in my diagnosis. Yes, I am open to the spiritual realm. Yes, I am in search of a deeper meaning in life.* If you answered yes to most of the questions above, you fit into the category of factors associated with longer survival outcomes according to The Cunningham Study. If you answered no to some or all of the questions above, you may want to develop more openness and curiosity towards emotional roots to cancer, to the spiritual realm and towards developing a deeper purpose in life.

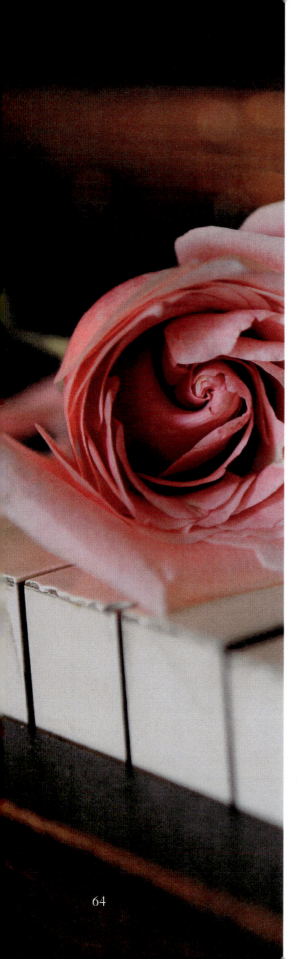

Section 2: Relationships Reflect Me: What Do You See?

Chapter 1

The Broken Heart

Let's take an assessment of where you are at relationally so that we can find out how you can improve your relational connections:

- Have you ever experienced a broken heart? What happened?

- Have you ever lost a significant relationship to death, divorce or separation?
  How did it impact you and is it resolved now?

- How are your relationships on a scale of 1 to 10? *(10 being the best relationships of your life and 1 being the worse relationships of your life)* Why?

- Are you able to be your true and authentic self with 1-3 people? Who are they and why or why not?

- Do you protect yourself emotionally and stop yourself from feeling deep, vulnerable emotions like sadness, depression, fear, loneliness, hopelessness, rejection or disappointment?

- How do you protect yourself from emotional pain and rejection and when did you start trying to protect yourself?

- Did you grow up with your parents saying things like "shame on you" when you did something wrong?

- What were your interactions with your parents like?

- Draw a picture of how your family related with each other and with you. Draw a picture of how you fit into your family.

- Reflect on your picture. What do you notice? Any new insights or emotions? *If strong emotions were evoked, I would recommend going through* **Chapter 3: Freeing Your Mind From Imprints of Trauma** *to process the image of your family using a memory or the image itself like you did to redesign your traumatic memories.*

- Do you value honesty and emotional vulnerability with your closest friends? Or do you keep everyone at a distance, including yourself? Why?

- Who are the top 5 people who have hurt you the most in life?

- What happened and what did they do to you?

- Is there still lingering emotional pain?

- Did you stop opening up to people after your experiences with these relationships?

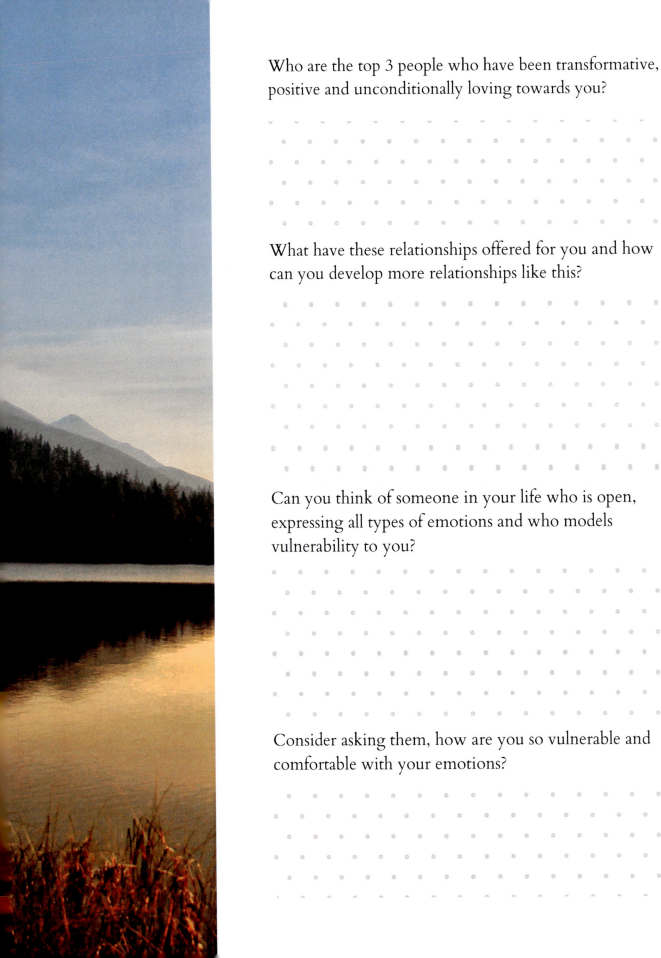

Who are the top 3 people who have been transformative, positive and unconditionally loving towards you?

What have these relationships offered for you and how can you develop more relationships like this?

Can you think of someone in your life who is open, expressing all types of emotions and who models vulnerability to you?

Consider asking them, how are you so vulnerable and comfortable with your emotions?

Let's look at a few strategies to increase your output of oxytocin by increasing social interactions. Here are some ways to increase your production of oxytocin:

- Physical contact such as hugs, massages, being intimate, shaking hands and breastfeeding
- Essential oils — Studies suggest that certain essential oils like clary sage oil may increase the production of oxytocin
- Making eye contact
- Laughing
- Throwing parties and having friends over for dinner
- Giving and receiving gifts
- Petting a dog, cat or other pet
- Doing "loving kindness" meditation or visualization
- Telling someone you love them
- Listening to calming music
- Speaking to a friend or family member on the phone
- Walking or exercising with someone
- Looking at photos or videos of people you care about

Pick 4-5 strategies in this list that you most connect with. Write down your strategies that you will implement on a daily or weekly basis:

_____
_____
_____
_____

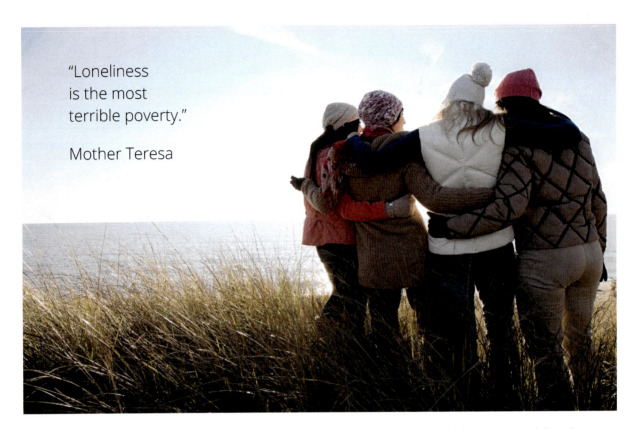

"Loneliness is the most terrible poverty."

Mother Teresa

Do you avoid talking to strangers or people you meet at public venues like the grocery store or the coffee shop? Why or why not?

Can you try to make small, micro-connections on a daily basis with people you meet throughout your day?

EXTRA JOURNALING & DRAWING SPACE

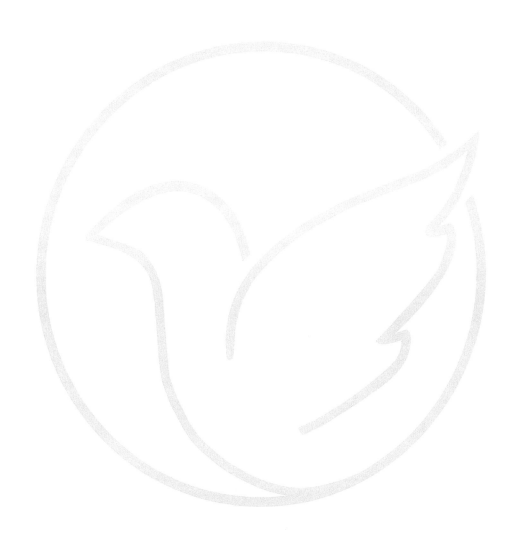

"Assumptions are the termites of relationships."
~Henry Winkler

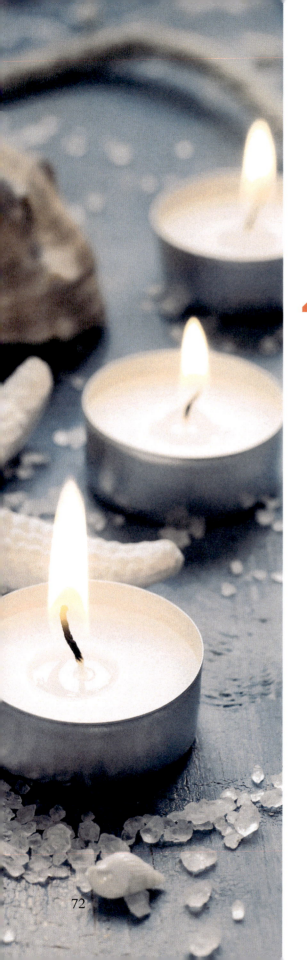

Section 2: Relationships Reflect Me: What Do You See?

Chapter 2

My Soul Deserves Peace

Create your own Loving-Kindness study. Engage in this study for 6 weeks. Every day, spend a few minutes meditating and thinking about friends and family members, saying the following over them:

"May you feel safe, may you feel happy, may you feel healthy and may you live with ease."

Record your daily and weekly interactions with strangers, friends and family.
How many interactions do you currently have on a daily and weekly basis?

How can you increase the number of social interactions that you have?

How can you increase the quality of your social interactions?

> I will give you a few ideas to see what fits your personality. I love to write letters to people to encourage them. I do this probably once a month or every few months and give it to someone who needs encouragement. I try to focus on their good qualities and what I love about them. I also like to interact with strangers in the grocery store, at the coffee shop or while I am on a walk. In fact, this is why my husband sometimes complains about going grocery shopping with me. Also, my husband and I love to have dinner parties and try to do them once a month as a way to stay socially connected.

What do you like to do?

Do you like to write cards to people? Do you like to throw parties?

Can you do this more often?

How do you know if you are struggling with bitterness?

First of all, if you feel anger and resentment every time you see someone, you have lingering bitterness and need to forgive. If you repeat the memories of hurt and betrayal over and over again in your mind, you probably need to forgive. If you find yourself not trusting people or shutting people out, you may need to forgive.

How do you know if you are easily offended?

Offense sounds like this:

1. Someone makes a decision that you don't agree with and moves forward. Or someone does or doesn't do something that you expect of them.

2. Internally, you wonder, why are they doing that or why did they NOT do this? If I were he or she, I would have made this decision or I would have done this….In these thoughts, there is an attitude of "I am right and they are wrong" and "I can't believe what they just did or said to me."

3. Internally, you may also be thinking, "They don't care about me or they don't notice that I need help."

4. I'm offended that they would do it this way, or not do this or make a decision that hurts me. They are wrong and I don't want to understand their perspective. I don't even want to talk about it.

EXAMPLE OF HOW TO AVOID OFFENSE:

We were planning a trip with friends and my husband wanted to invite a family member. As the dates got closer, we started to plan more details and shared with our friends that we were planning on bringing a family member.

A few weeks prior to the trip, one of our friends asked us why we were bringing our family member. In addition, they mentioned that they had a separate conversation with our mutual friend about why it wasn't a good idea. We were unaware that this conversation happened and felt hurt that we were not included in it.

Our friend continued the conversation and brought up several reasons why it wouldn't make sense for the purpose of the trip to bring our family member. There were other things brought into the conversation that were unrelated. I left that conversation feeling very hurt and misunderstood.

I easily could have taken offense.

Instead, I chose to forgive my friends every day for a week when the bitterness surfaced.

> Secondly, I tried to see the situation from my friend's perspective.

Further, I wrote down some of my thoughts about the conversation and things that I wanted to bring up in a conversation with my friends. I planned a time to talk to them about how I was feeling.

A week after the conversation, we had a Zoom call with everyone involved. I shared my hurt, frustration and perspective of what happened. I felt heard in the conversation and affirmed in my perspective. I then was able to hear the perspective of everyone involved. After this interaction, I was able to let the situation go and agree that it may be best for us to keep it a friend trip.

I avoided taking offense by:
1. Choosing forgiveness.
2. Opening up a conversation to discuss my perspective and to hear the other perspectives.
3. Integrated different perspectives with my own perspective and found the ability to put myself in each of my friend's shoes.
4. Staying humble enough to realize that I could be wrong and it wasn't "my way or the highway."
5. Choosing not to judge someone for his or her perspective or his or her approach in communication.

> In the end, our conversations allowed the relationships to become stronger instead of weaker and allowed a deeper sense of understanding for everyone involved.

Do you find that you take offense easily in relationships?

When have you taken offense in relationships? Explain a situation that you remember.

Can you think of an offense that is still lingering that has caused a rift in your relationships?

Do you make it a habit in relationships to seek understanding by asking questions when you need to clarify motives and thoughts behind an action or conversation? Why or why not?

Do you believe that bitterness is impacting your physical body in a negative way?

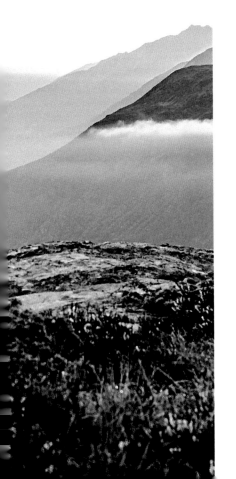

Do you believe that offense is impacting your physical body in a negative way?

EXTRA JOURNALING & DRAWING SPACE

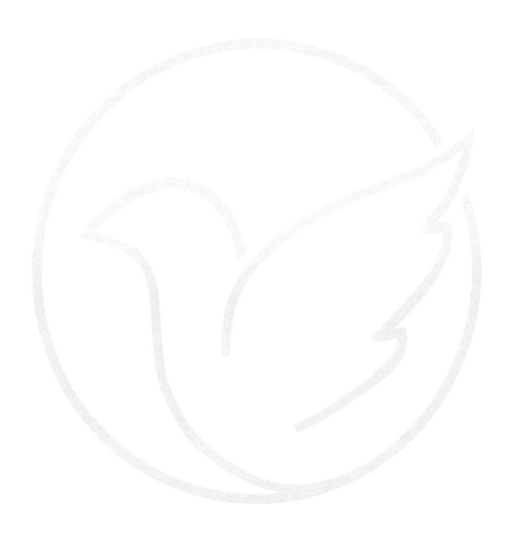

"Wise men speak because they have something to say, fools because they have to say something."
~Plato

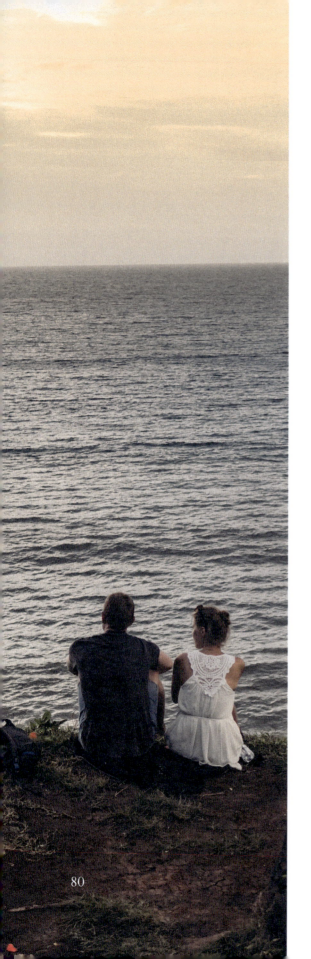

Section 2: Relationships Reflect Me: What Do You See?

Chapter 3

Into Me You See

In the first step, we work to uncover critical thoughts about yourself, your partner and your relationship. If you are not in a romantic relationship, you can do this exercise on a friendship or a relationship with a family member.

If you struggle to access your negative thought patterns, you may be using substances or addictive habits to suppress your awareness of thought patterns and emotional patterns. We can use alcohol, drugs, food, TV, exercise, video games, pornography, smoking or other habits to suppress our thoughts and emotions.

Try an experiment. Stop all addictive behaviors and habits for 2 weeks and try to allow your true thoughts and feelings to arise. Continue as you begin to better connect with yourself, grow in emotional intelligence and work to rewire your brain.

Any early defensive patterns or attachment patterns that we develop in childhood can limit us when we relate to close relationships as adults. Based upon this chapter, which attachment style did you develop with your parents when you were growing up? Secure, anxious, avoidant or disorganized? Why?

Which attachment style do you tend to develop in romantic relationships? Secure, dismissive-avoidant, anxious-preoccupied or fearful-avoidant?
How do you notice this attachment pattern?

Do you struggle to share vulnerable emotions with men? Why?

How were you raised in regards to self-expression and emotional expression? Did people in your family freely express their emotions with each other? Why or why not?

Do you have memories where you were deeply hurt and rejected? Did this change your way of relating with others?

Do you want to have authentic, vulnerable relationships again?

> If you do have a memory that you felt shamed, hurt or rejected, let's work through that memory now using the steps in **Chapter 3: Freeing Your Mind From Imprints of Trauma.**

EXTRA JOURNALING & DRAWING SPACE

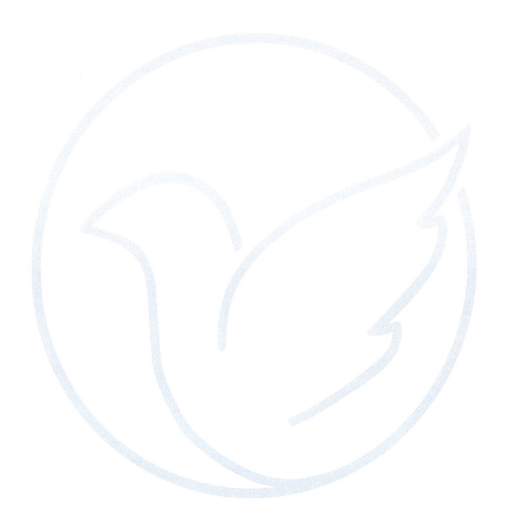

"Be kinder than necessary,
for everyone you meet is fighting some kind of battle."
~*Anonymous*

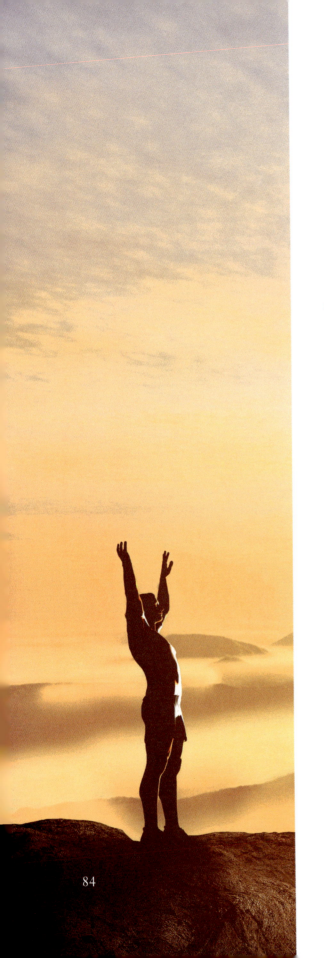

Section 2: Relationships Reflect Me: What Do You See?

Chapter 4

Come Out Of Hiding

When was the first time that you remember feeling shame?

Did you start to hide your true sense of self for a false sense of self? Explain.

Write down all of the memories from your past that you felt a deep sense of shame, remorse or regret:

What is your true sense of self that you hide from people?

What is your false sense of self that you present to the world to hide the shame that you feel sometimes?

What interferes with true intimacy in your relationships?

Let's do an exercise on integrity and integration of the external and the internal self:

What are the words that you would use to describe your **internal self** (the one that you only know and interact with)?

What are the words that you would use to describe your **external self** (the one the world sees and interacts with)?

Now, put 2 chairs facing each other and sit in one chair that represents your internal self. How does it feel to sit there?

How old do you feel and why?

Sit in the chair opposite the chair that represents your internal self and examine how it feels to be your external self. How do you feel?

How old are you and why?

We have internal strategies to defend against intimacy and vulnerability, especially when we have been hurt. Many times people will create the internal habit of retreating from intimacy through isolation.

We tend to justify it by thinking or saying, "I need space. I need time alone to chill. I'm too busy. I'm too stressed. I'm too tired."

The defensive strategy to isolate is mainly unconscious and not something we consciously plan. We can develop core beliefs in our subconscious mind that promote isolation and withdrawal from relationships out of the fear of emotional pain.

Isolation is different from time spent in self-contemplation, constructive planning or solitude. Isolation promotes an increase in critical thoughts towards yourself, your partner and leads to self-destructive behaviors. A good way to view isolation is that patterns of isolation promote carelessness towards your emotional well-being.

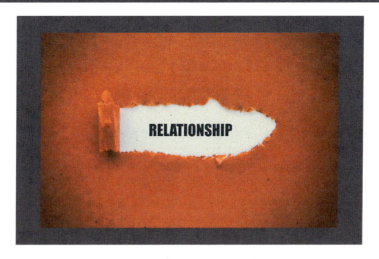

Ask the following questions of yourself to understand further:

Have I been isolating myself lately? Why?

Do I have a tendency to isolate myself? Why?

Did I spend a lot of time alone as a child? Why?

When I am alone, how do I spend my time?

Do I have healthy inward habits or critical inward habits? Why?

Do I tend to choose isolated activities over being social? Why?

[Some people will react against being vulnerable by attempting to control their partner to maintain distance. Some may become authoritarian, condescending with verbal threats that involve rejection or abandonment of their partner.]

Are there any obvious ways in which I am controlling towards my partner, friends or family members?

Why do I try to control?

Can I be punishing when things don't go my way? Why?

Do I withdraw affection or act cold if I don't get my way? Why?

Do I play the victim?

Do I allow my spouse to control me? Why?

Be a curious observer of your interactions with your significant other. Try to identify specific patterns or fights that occur in your relationship on a regular basis. When you feel intense emotions that spark a fight, reflect on that fight and try to find the deeper belief that sparked that interaction. Let's start with identifying one negative pattern in your relationship.

//

What negative pattern do you see in your relationship with your significant other?

What thought patterns are emerging that are critical towards you?

What thoughts are you noticing that are negative towards your partner?

What thoughts are you noticing that are negative towards your relationship?

If you are struggling to find any patterns in your relationship, write about the details of your last fight that tends to be a reoccurring fight:

What are your critical thought patterns about your relationship before and after this fight:

What are the emotions that you feel before and during this fight?

Now concentrate on these emotions while you close your eyes. Have a pen in your hand and be ready to write. While you concentrate on these emotions, follow your emotions back to a memory that feels the same. What memory appears in your conscious mind as you concentrate on these emotions?

What conclusion did you come to about others, the spiritual world or yourself in that memory? How did that memory impact you?

I had to confront the maladaptive belief that I held after judging traditional roles in my parent's marriage. My belief that I developed as a child sounded something like this:

> "I never want to be a stay-at-home wife or mother. I want my life to be significant and have a major impact on the world. Being a stay-at-home wife and mother will not allow me to have a significant contribution to the world."

This was my perception of reality and the perception was not serving me well anymore. I needed to confront this belief to change my patterns in my marriage. I was stuck on autopilot and literally could not do anything that remotely looked like a task that a traditional wife or mother would do on a day-to-day basis because of this maladaptive core belief.

Once I had awareness of my unhealthy pattern and where it was coming from, confronting this belief and pattern became easy. After I confessed and apologized to my husband with the letter I had written, I also needed to confront the maladaptive core belief directly.

My verbal confrontation went something like this:

"You have not been prioritizing your relationship with your husband. You believe that you cannot be a wife, mother and a businesswoman. You are stuck in the belief that you have to choose between the three roles instead of doing all of these roles at the same time. As a child, you watched your mom and dad and you judged their relationship. That was wrong.

This belief that you created based upon a judgment is not helping you. In fact, you are sabotaging your marriage right now. It was wrong for you to judge your mom for deciding to be a stay-at-home mom. It was her choice and she did it out of love for you.

You are very selfish and critical of others when their life choices don't align with your perspective. You need to release the judgment that you made against your mother and allow yourself to step into your role as a mother and a wife so that your family life can flourish."

Now that you reviewed my example from the book and read my process of confrontation, do you have clarity on how this process goes? What pattern do you notice in your relationship that is unhealthy and perhaps sabotaging your relationship?

What maladaptive core belief from your childhood is connected to this unhealthy pattern in your relationship?

> If you are struggling to find a maladaptive core belief, reflect on your thoughts and emotions in your relationship.

What are the emotions that you feel on a regular basis with your partner?

Do you feel angry or critical towards your partner?

Do you feel abandoned after conflict?

Do your thoughts and emotions remind you of any relationships from childhood?

Is this how you were treated as a child?

Do you relate to your partner the way that your parents related to each other?

> Are you ready to confront this belief and the internal monologue that connects to this belief? If so, follow the next steps. You can choose to write a confrontation, confront yourself out loud or share the confrontation with a close friend.

What is the belief or internal monologue that you are discovering about yourself and your relationship with your partner that you want to confront now?

How can you confront your critical internal monologue that is hindering your relationship? You can write a confrontation here:

You may need to confront your belief by apologizing and admitting to your significant other any pattern that you have in your relationship that hinders intimacy. What would you say to your significant other now after reflecting upon your relationship?

Finally, it is time to work on the behavior that needs to change. After you confront critical thought patterns and the maladaptive core belief, you will be free to change the behavioral patterns. Be specific in what behavior you are going to stop doing and what behavior you are going to begin doing.

I decided to stop working when my husband came home from work and either cook for us before he got home or cook dinner together. Each day, I made sure that we had a meal together before I went back to work in my office again.

What behavior change can you decide to make today?

_____

After you change your behavior, carry out the new behaviors on a daily basis and progressively add in new behaviors as you succeed in the beginning changes. Every action based upon the awareness of the beliefs that you are confronting either strengthens or weakens the connections in the brain.

New actions performed over and over again build and strengthen new neural connections in the brain.

What other new behaviors would you like to add in?

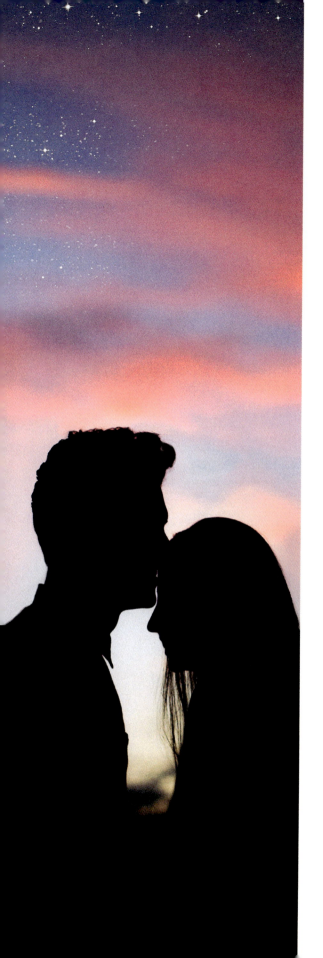

Section 2: Relationships Reflect Me: What Do You See?

Chapter 5

The Art of Developing True Intimacy

"The most empowering relationships are those in which each partner lifts the other to a higher possession of their own being."
~Pierre Teilhard de Chardin

Try a month fast from gossip...

...where you decide not to talk about other people when they are not present or where you do not engage when other people are gossiping.

To diffuse gossip, you can learn to say the following phrases after someone shares intimate details about someone:

- "Perhaps we should discuss this next time when we are with Becky so that she can tell us what happened."

- "I think that we should give Becky the benefit of the doubt."

- "I will never forget how Becky made a meal for me after my son died, it was so generous and kind of her."

"Watch the little things; a small leak will sink a great ship." ~Benjamin Franklin

To move from a cliché relationship to a more intimate relationship, do this exercise with your partner:

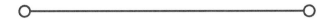

Pull two chairs close to each other to the point where you are holding hands and your knees are touching. Take 3 minutes each to share personal facts about your life and who you are. Reveal yourself to your partner in a new way.

While in this intimate moment, ask the following questions and both you and your partner give answers:

- Which of your dreams got lost along the way when I was too busy pursuing my own dreams?

- How can I better support you in the pursuit of your dreams?

- Do you know what you want your life to look like long-term?

- Are you able to share your dreams wtih me?

- Have I been supportive of your dreams or have I been judgmental and harsh towards your dreams?

- Have you let go of some of your dreams because of practical things or an inability to know how to move forward?

- What is our dream that we want to accomplish together?

Examine the following questions about your relationship together and separately:

What is the purpose of your relationship?

Do you have a vision for your lives together as a couple and how can you define the purpose of your relationship together?

How can you help your partner to become the best version of him or herself? (If you don't have a partner, you can focus on another relationship like a family member or best friend)

How can I help my partner to fulfill their dreams?

What are your partner's needs and how can you help him or her to fulfill those needs?

Is your relationship your top priority? Why or why not?

> Do the following exercise on complaining and gratitude:

Attempt to go 24-hours without any complaints at all. Record what you complain about each time. Were you able to complete 24-hours without any complaints at all?

Did you complain about your significant other?

Write a gratitude list:

I'm thankful for:
1) The following people, 2) The following things, 3) Specifics/others

[
A note on gratitude's: It is best to be specific. Instead of saying, I'm grateful to be alive, be more specific. I'm grateful for the rainbow that I saw today. I'm grateful that my husband made my favorite meal tonight. After writing a very specific gratitude list, read your gratitude list 4 times in 24-hours, after lunch, before dinner, before going to bed and before going to school or work.
]

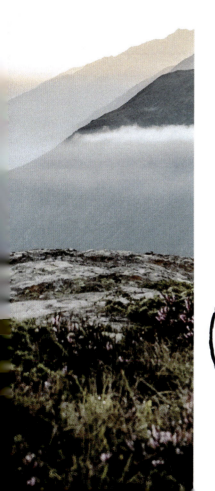

How do you feel after completing this exercise?

> When we focus on what is right instead of what is wrong in our lives, our attitude improves.

The next step is to make a list of all the things you are thankful for in your significant other and mail a copy to them (even if they live with you).

Take 5 minutes to give the deepest, most intimate hug to your partner. You can put on meditative music and have essential oils diffusing in the room. As you hug, notice your partner's breath and heartbeat. You will begin to feel their vulnerability at the same time that you begin to feel oneness in your bodies.

Pick one topic that you know that you disagree on and decide to have a lively discussion with ground rules. Create the following ground rules around the conversation:

1. No name-calling.
2. Show respect and kindness.
3. No judgment or sarcasm.
4. Try to be a curious observer to understand why your partner came to the conclusion that they carry about the given topic.
5. The job of each person at the end is to be able to summarize what the person thinks about the subject and why he or she came to that conclusion.
6. Find one area of common ground in the subject, where you agree with the other person and talk about this.

Write down what you discovered about yourself and the other person here:

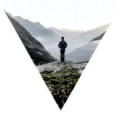

Exercise with significant other on hopes & dreams:

Buy a journal to share with your partner where you both write dreams for the future. If you don't have a partner, you can buy a journal for yourself and do this exercise.

My top 3 dreams for my life:

....

....

....

What do you want to see 5 years from now & 10 years from now?

What dreams intersect for both you and your partner?

What do you want to do together?

What dreams does your partner have that are different than yours?

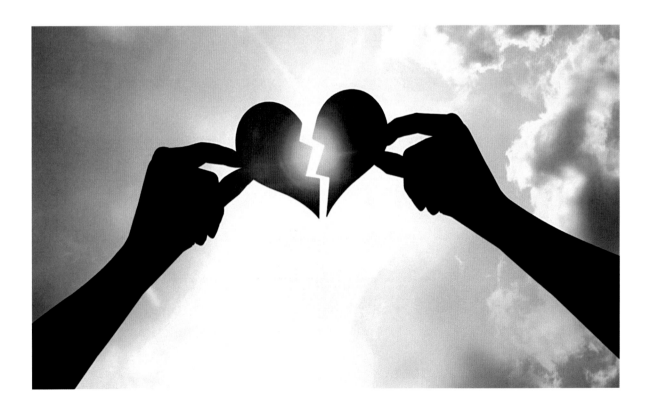

How can you help make their dreams happen?

What are 3 practical steps you can focus on for the next 6 months that will help contribute to your 5 year vision of what you want to see manifest in your life?

....
....
....
....
....
....
....

Exercise with significant other:
Greatest Disappointment in
Life Now & in the Past

Date Night

Set a date night to eat at a private location where you can talk with your significant other. If you have not shared your greatest disappointment with him or her, plan to do so on the date. Try not to make the greatest disappointment about them, like "my greatest disappointment was marrying you."

Instead, focus on a disappointment that has nothing to do with your significant other. Ask them what their greatest disappointment is from the past and what their greatest disappointment is now. Focus on listening intently and drawing out their intimate thoughts and emotions.

Show empathy, love & support.

Ask this:
How can I help you to overcome this disappointment?

Do you feel closer to your partner now?

Did you learn something new about your partner or yourself?

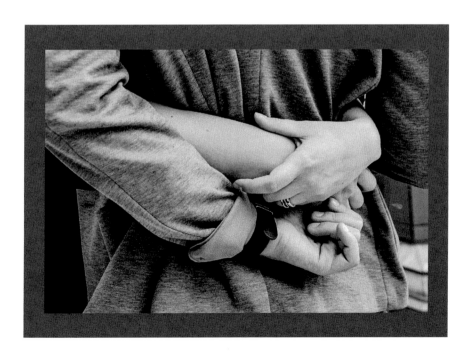

Section 3: Unraveling the Imprint of Trauma

Chapter 1

The Dream-Like State of Surviving Trauma & How to Move Past Surviving into Thriving

1. When you read this chapter of *Braving The Storm*, which part of the chapter spoke to you the most and why?

2. Without thinking too hard about it, draw the most traumatic thing that has ever happened to you.

What do you see in the drawing that you were not aware of previously?

3. Do you have unresolved trauma that you are consciously aware of?
   If the answer is yes, write down the unresolved trauma and why it still remains unresolved. If the answer is no, is it possible that you have unresolved trauma that you are not consciously aware of? Are you open and curious to find out?

4. Have you ever experienced symptoms of Post-traumatic Stress Disorder or PTSD?

[
Symptoms occur after trauma and include: flashbacks, headaches, backaches, anxiety, depression, living in a dream-like state, on heightened alert, learning is near impossible, lack of ability to cope with daily stressors, lack of ability to focus or tunnel vision, use of drugs and alcohol in an attempt to cope, a lack of purpose and trouble sleeping.
]

Which symptoms did you experience or are you still experiencing?

What was the traumatic event that triggered PTSD for you?

If you are numb as you write about the traumatic event, try this: draw a picture of the traumatic event that triggered PTSD symptoms for you.

What do you notice in this drawing that you were not aware of previously?

If you have new traumatic memories coming up for you, go back to **Chapter 3: Freeing Your Mind From Imprints Of Trauma** *to do the memory work steps.*

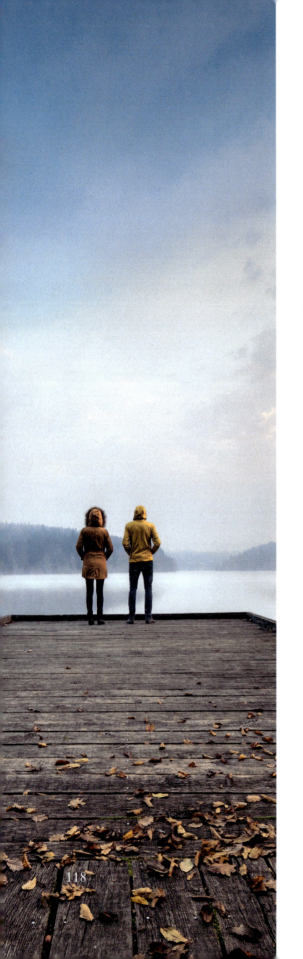

Section 3: Unraveling the Imprint of Trauma

Chapter 2

**Mindfulness:
Ending The Phantom Existence**

What in this chapter resonated the most with you? Why?

Open yourself up to your inner experience by declaring the following out loud, **"In the past, I have chosen to numb, ignore and suppress my emotions because of fear, I now choose to open up my mind and my body to feeling again so that I can resolve my past fully."**

Start a journaling process to help connect your physical sensations to your emotions. Let's try some free association journaling. You can start with your current thoughts or start writing about an object in front of you. Dump your thoughts without editing or judging them.

As you write your thoughts, you may notice changes in your physical body as emotions begin to manifest. Try to write and describe what **physical sensations** you notice in this process.

Do you feel pressure or heat?

Are you struggling to breathe?

If so, let's try some breathing exercises. Focus on your breath. Take a deep breath in and out. Tap your chest below your collarbone. Deliberately take a few slow, deep breaths.

Pay attention until the very end of the out breath and wait a moment before you inhale again. As you continue to breathe, notice the air moving in and out of your lungs. Think about the role oxygen plays in bathing your tissues with the energy that you need to feel alive.

Do you feel a tightening of your chest, muscular tension, tingling or a caving in feeling?

Do you feel a hollow, uncomfortable, gnawing feeling in your belly?

Allow your mind to focus on the sensations in your body.

Notice how your bodily sensations change based upon the movement of your body, how you breathe and what you are thinking about.

What do you notice currently about your bodily sensations?

Practice labeling the physical sensations that you are noticing...
When I feel my chest tighten, my breathing restricted, my thoughts racing, I am feeling anxious.
At the core of recovery from trauma is self-awareness.

What do you notice now?

What happens next?

What are you thinking about when you feel anxious?

> "Mirror neurons allow for syncing with another person in a relationship. When people are in sync with one another, they will sit or stand in a similar manner and their voices will take on the same rhythms."
>
> "When someone has experienced trauma, boundaries were crossed that caused the person to not feel seen, heard or mirrored. When boundaries are crossed, mirror neurons can be misappropriated and now the very thing that allows us to sync with others relationally can make us vulnerable to being overtaken by another person's internal experience."

Consider the 2 quotes above while answering the following questions:

1. Do you find it difficult or easy to mirror people around you?

2. Whom in your life have you most easily been able to sync within a relationship? Why?

3. Do you find yourself chronically out of sync with people around you? Why?

4. Do you tend to take on other people's emotions? Has unresolved trauma caused you to have poorly defined boundaries?

EXTRA JOURNALING & DRAWING SPACE

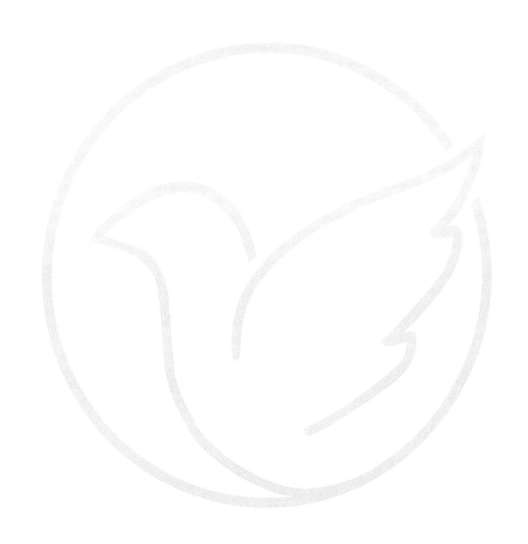

"Whereever you are, be all there."
~Jim Elliot

> "Trauma will increase the risk of misinterpreting whether a situation is dangerous or safe. Faulty alarms from trauma lead a person to either blow up or shut down."

Do you struggle to interpret whether a situation is dangerous or safe? Why or why not?

Have you now or in the past struggled with either blowing up in anger or shutting down in relational exchanges and slight conflict? Why?

"Mindfulness is the ability to hover calmly and objectively over thoughts and emotions, taking our time to respond to relational interactions and experiences."

How well are you able to hover calmly and objectively over your thoughts and emotions?

Are you able to take your time in responding to relational interactions? Why or why not?

Do you often feel hijacked by emotions, swept away into a panic attack or utter despair?

Explain a recent time when you were hijacked by your emotions. What happened?

> "The only way that we can change how we feel is by becoming aware of our inner experience and learning to befriend what is going on inside of ourselves."

Have you befriended what is going on inside of yourself? Why or why not?

Try to look at the most recent time that you were overtaken by intense emotions in a relational interaction. Spend some time reflecting on why this happened. Close your eyes, focus on the relational exchange and answer the following questions:

What are you noticing internally?

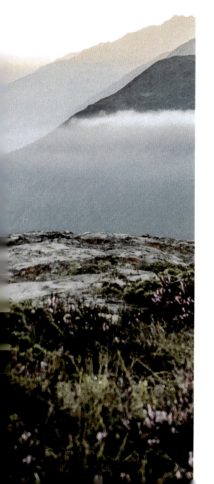

What emotions are you feeling?

Is there another time in your life that you felt this way? When?

If a new memory comes up for you, go back to **Chapter 3: Freeing Your Mind From Imprints Of Trauma** *to go through the process of redesigning this memory.*

Here are a few strategies to pick from to grow in the ability to be self-aware and befriend internal sensations:

- **Rhythmic movements such as dancing.** Can you join a dance group or a dance class?

- Can you schedule regular massages to reconnect with your physical body?

- **Find other ways to move:** Can you join a Pilates class, try a new sport, go to a kickboxing class, run or join a class to learn self-defense?

- Journaling: Have you committed to a process of journaling to help grow in mindfulness?

- **Meditation:** Can you try to incorporate this to help with mindfulness?

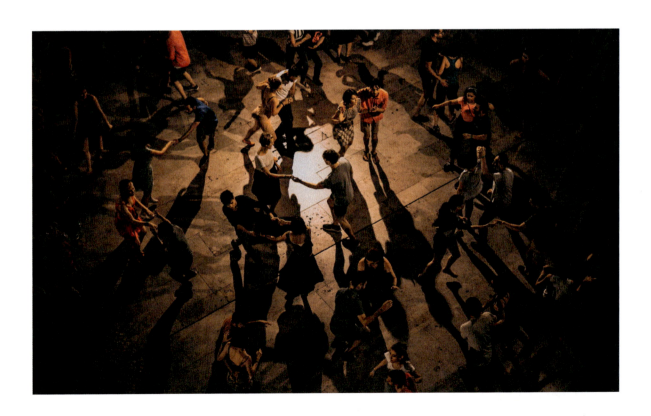

If a person was running towards you with a knife, how would you feel?

Did you answer with an action that you would perform like, "I would jump out of the way?" Or did you answer with an emotion, "I would be very scared?"

If you answered with an action that you would perform, you may be suffering from alexithymia because of trauma.

> "People with alexithymia substitute action words for emotional language. Someone with alexithymia registers emotions as physical problems instead of signals that need their attention. Someone with alexithymia continually suppresses their emotions and is almost completely unable to express their emotions."

Do you think that you have alexithymia?

Do you want to reconnect with your emotions and learn to reconnect with yourself after trauma? Why or why not?

Have you experienced symptoms like migraine headaches, asthma attacks, chronic back and neck pain, fibromyalgia, digestive problems, chronic fatigue, which do not have a clear biological basis?

> "Researchers discovered that some people experience the loss of self after trauma. Paul Schilder, a German psychoanalyst found that the depersonalized individual experiences the world in a dream-like state. They have become complete strangers to themselves and live a phantom existence. In an attempt to control their lives, trauma victims ignore gut feelings and numb their awareness by learning to hide from themselves."

END THE PHANTOM EXISTENCE...

Have you become a stranger to yourself after trauma?

Do you hide from yourself?

Are you ready to stop hiding from yourself and heal from past trauma? Why or why not?

Develop your emotional intelligence by practicing discerning the emotional expressions of others. Look at the following pictures of emotions, what emotions are being expressed?

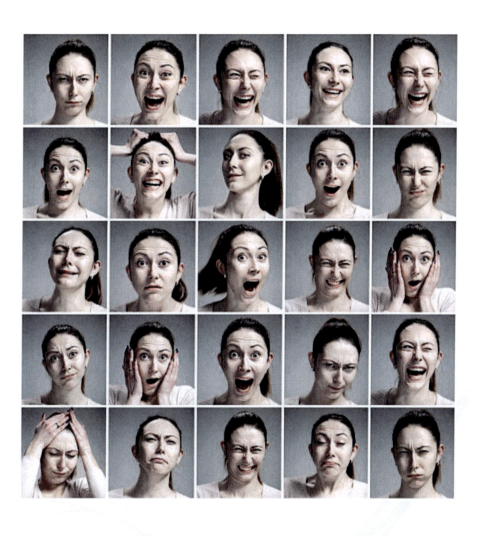

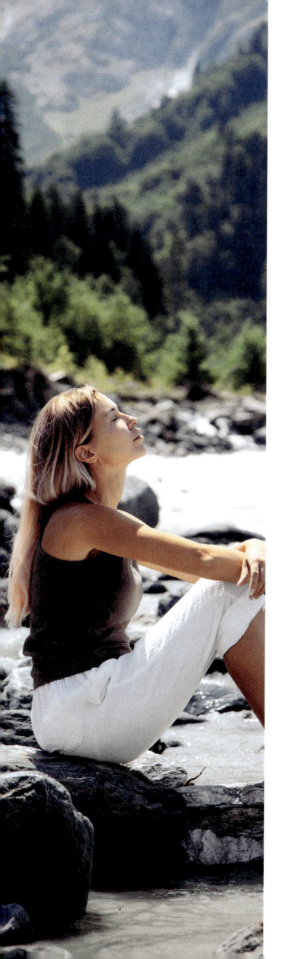

Section 3: Unraveling the Imprint of Trauma

Chapter 3

Become a Curious Observer of Your Internal World & Own Your Emotional Brain

What spoke to you the most from this chapter? Why?

Take this quiz to find our your ACE, childhood trauma score:

While you were growing up, during your first 18 years of life:

1. Did a parent or other adult in the household often or very often...   Yes _____
Swear at you, insult you, put you down or humiliate you? **OR**   No _____
Act in a way that made you afraid that you might be physically hurt?

2. Did a parent or other adult in the household often or very often...   Yes _____
Push, grab, slap or throw something at you? **OR**   No _____
Ever hit you so hard that you had marks or were injured?

3. Did an adult or person at least 5 years older than you ever...   Yes _____
Touch or fondle you or have you touch their body in a sexual way?   No _____
OR
Attempt or actually have oral, anal or vaginal intercourse with you?

4. Did you often or very often feel that ... No one in your family   Yes _____
loved you or thought you were important or special? **OR**   No _____
Your family didn't look out for each other, feel close to each other
or support each other?

5. Did you often or very often feel that ...You didn't have enough to   Yes _____
eat, had to wear dirty clothes and had no one to protect you? **OR**   No _____
Your parents were too drunk or high to take care of you or take you
to the doctor if you needed it?

6. Were your parents ever separated or divorced? Yes _____ No _____

7. Was your mother or stepmother: Yes _____
Often or very often pushed, grabbed, slapped or had something No _____
thrown at her? **OR** Sometimes, often or very often kicked, bitten,
hit with a fist or hit with something hard? **OR** Ever repeatedly hit
for at least a few minutes or threatened with a gun or knife?

8. Did you live with anyone who was a problem drinker, alcoholic Yes _____
or using street drugs? No _____

9. Was a household member depressed, mentally ill or did a household Yes _____
member attempt suicide? No _____

10. Did a household member go to prison? Yes _____
 No _____

Now add up your **"Yes"** answers: _____ This is your ACE Score.
In order to interpret the meaning of your ACE score, review pages
226-229 in *Braving The Storm* to better understand your results.

Adapted from: http://www.acestudy.org/files/ACE_Score_Calculator.pdf

Change begins when we learn to own our emotional brain. We can learn to observe and tolerate physical sensations in our body, while we develop the ability to verbalize and express a wide-range of emotions. Start now by committing yourself to be a curious observer of your internal world. Decide to stop suppressing bodily sensations and emotions.

Can you think of anyone whom you felt safe with growing up? Who?

Think about that relationship and journal about your relationship with him or her. How did you feel when you were in that person's presence?

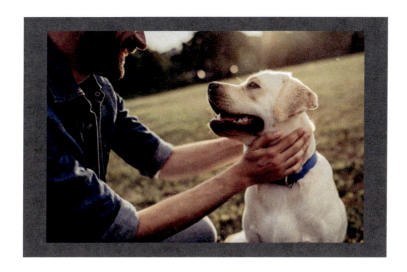

What did you share with them?

Can you imagine yourself connecting with another person in that same way? Why or why not?

If you don't remember feeling safe with anyone, when you were young, engaging with horse or dogs would be safer and helpful at reestablishing basic trust. Do you like animals?

Do you own a dog or a cat?

Unresolved trauma from childhood affects relationships long-term until we resolve the trauma and restore our ability to trust and synchronize with another human being. People with a history of trauma, abuse and neglect struggle to open up and many times end up sabotaging relationships in their lives.

Do you tend to sabotage the close relationships in your life? How? Why?

Do you struggle to open up your deepest thoughts and emotions to those closest to you because of a fear of rejection and fear of betrayal?

Imagine what you were like when you were a newborn: Were you loveable and full of spunk?

Draw a family portrait. What did your family look like growing up? Draw it just as you felt when you were growing up and just as your family members were without any judgment or editing.

After you draw your family portrait, journal about your family portrait for 15-minutes per day for 4 days. What do you notice about your role in the family and where you are positioned in the family portrait?

What do you notice about your family portrait?

How do you feel when you look at your family portrait?

What memories surface consciously when you look at the family portrait?

What is the most stressful, terrifying memory that you can remember based upon looking at your family portrait?

How did you feel in that memory?

How did that memory impact your life and who you are today?

What would you say to yourself after you endured that experience?

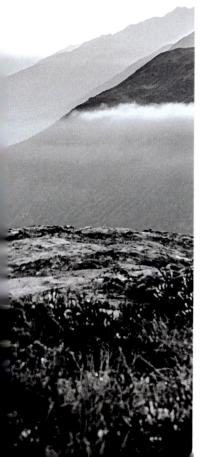

Have you worked through the memories in **Chapter 3: Freeing Your Mind From Imprints Of Trauma**?

Read the following excerpt from the book:

> "If someone is held down, trapped or prevented from taking effective action during trauma, they are at risk for developing PTSD (Post-traumatic Stress Disorder) at the same time that the body continues in a state of fight or flight."

Have you ever been in a traumatic situation that you could not easily escape from? For example, a domestically violent relationship, child abuse or a car accident. Explain.

"*When trauma victims can physically experience what it would have felt like to fight back or run away, they can relax, smile and feel a sense of completion. The self-defense treatment approach can teach women or men to recondition the freeze response by learning to transform fear into positive fighting energy.*"

Can you engage in the strategies that we mentioned in the book, *Braving The Storm,* in order to engage the body to feel a sense of completion with past trauma? Some of the strategies include kickboxing, self-defense classes and running.

• •

"Research has found that those with a history of childhood sexual and physical abuse have a higher risk of repeated suicide attempts and self-cutting. Patients, who did not improve, had no memories of feeling safe with anyone during their childhood. If someone carries a memory and feeling of safety with just one person, the bond and feeling of safety can be reactivated with another adult and trauma can be addressed more readily. "

Have you ever tried to commit suicide? Describe what happened.

Did you use self-cutting as a way to express emotions that you couldn't figure out how to express?

Do you have a history of childhood sexual and physical abuse that you are aware of?

U*se* **Chapter 3: Freeing Your Mind From Imprints Of Trauma** *to help with memory work if you have memories of childhood sexual and physical abuse that need to be resolved.*

In childhood, did you experience any chronically stressful events that caused you to numb your emotions? What happened?

Do you still have a tendency to numb or suppress your emotions?

Can you decide to stop numbing and grow in mindfulness of your emotions? If so, say this out loud with me, **"During childhood, I started the habit of numbing my emotions in order to survive because of the chronic stress of _____.
I forgive my family and _____
because my soul deserves peace. I also make a new decision to stop numbing my emotions and to start feeling again. I want to heal and I want to be whole. I don't want to numb and control my emotions any longer."**

How does that feel?

EXTRA JOURNALING & DRAWING SPACE

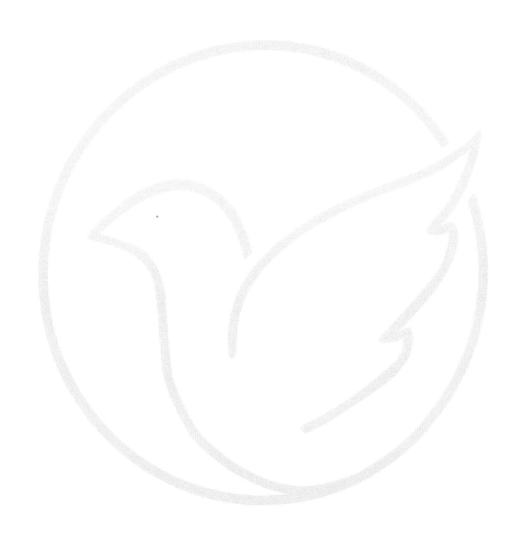

"Good timber does not grow with ease.
The stronger the wind, the stronger the trees."
~William Marriott

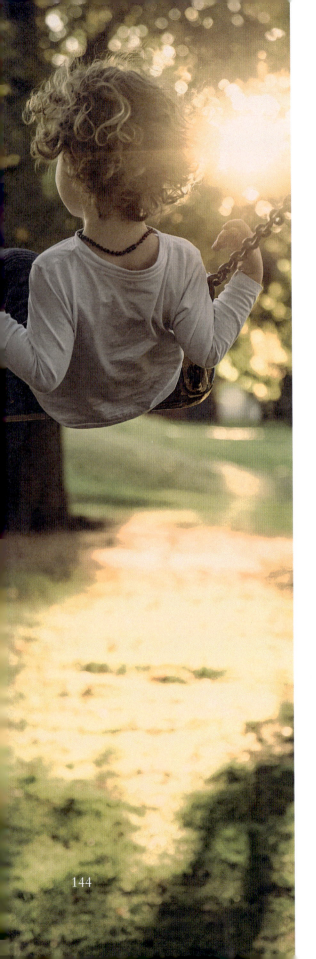

Section 3: Unraveling the Imprint of Trauma

Chapter 4

Reversing the Amnesia of Trauma to Fully Integrate Your Brain

What was the biggest thing that impacted you in this chapter and why?

> "Delayed recall of trauma and partial or complete amnesia can be common after trauma. In 19-38% of cases of childhood sexual abuse, the victims experienced total memory loss."

Have you ever recalled a memory that you didn't have access to for years because of the intensity of the trauma?

Is it possible that you have repressed memories because of trauma in your subconscious mind?

Now, let's do an exercise together. Without thinking too hard about it, draw a picture of a repressed memory that occurred for you in childhood that was so traumatic, the memory could not be integrated and stored in a normal manner. *If you don't have anything to draw, try this. Ask your subconscious mind, "Is there any repressed memory that I need to gain access to in order to heal?" Wait for an answer.*

What do you see in the picture?

If you have discovered a new memory that you need to process using our memory work exercise, go back to **Chapter 3: Freeing Your Mind From Imprints Of Trauma** *to work through this memory.*

Have you ever experienced an inability to fully recall a memory, but felt physical sensations, intense emotions and vivid images that don't make sense to your conscious brain? Explain.

With traumatic experiences that you recall, are you able to tell a coherent story or is it still fragmented in your conscious brain?

If you need to work on fully integrating any fragmented images, start by trying to draw the fragmented images that you see here:

What do you see? What is this correlated to?

What physical sensations and intense emotions do you feel time to time that you don't fully understand?

Now, follow these emotions and physical sensations back in your memory, does any memory or image appear in your mind? Describe.

If you have gained enough new information, try to work through the memory in **Chapter 3: Freeing Your Mind From Imprints Of Trauma.**

If at any time in this work that you are doing, you need help or you are being re-traumatized, reach out for professional help. You can reach out to Cancer Peace University for individual guidance or reach out to a trusted counselor trained in memory work.

Free writing can be an amazing tool to help access the inmost recesses of the heart and mind. Use any object as a way to enter into a stream of association. Look at the object and start writing whatever comes to your mind and follow your thoughts until you empty all of your thoughts on this paper.

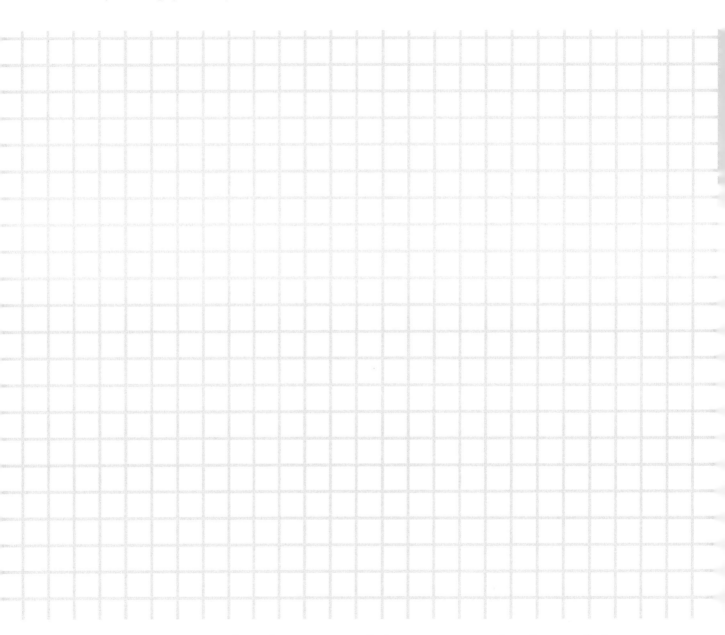

Once you empty your thoughts, you may feel an emotion. What do you feel? Why?

Now, take 4 days in a row to write for 15-minutes a day about the most traumatic, stressful thing that has ever happened to you that you have conscious recollection of.

If you are ever overcome with intense emotions during these exercises do the following:

Exercise 1:

If your chest tightens and breath almost disappears, focus on your hands. Move your hands and flex them so that they feel separate from the trauma.

Exercise 2:

Focus on your "out breath." Notice how you can change the flow of your breath while you focus on breathing in and out, in and out, breathing through intense emotions.

Exercise 3:

Feel the weight of your body. Plant your feet on the floor while you sit up straight. Next, tap your chest under your collarbone.

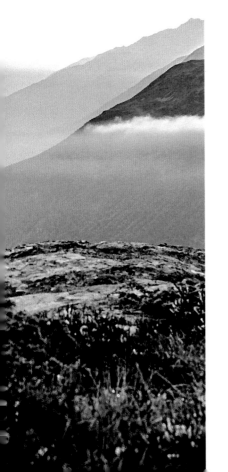

Day 1

How did you feel at the time of the most traumatic event in your life? Explain the details of what happened.

How do you feel now about the most traumatic thing that has ever happened to you?

How did this trauma impact your life?

Day 2

How did you feel at the time of the most traumatic event in your life? Explain in detail how you felt and why.

How do you feel now about the most traumatic thing that has ever happened to you?

How did this trauma impact your life?

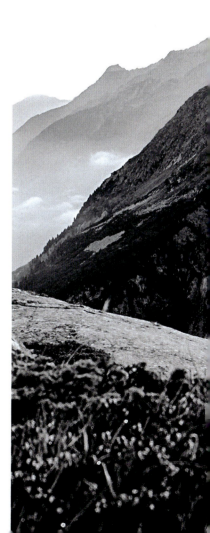

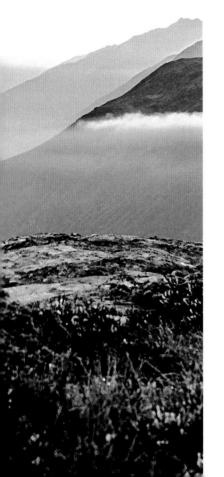

Day 3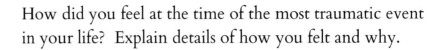

How did you feel at the time of the most traumatic event in your life? Explain details of how you felt and why.

How do you feel now about the most traumatic thing that has ever happened to you?

How did this trauma impact your life?

Day 4

How did you feel at the time of the most traumatic event in your life? Explain how you felt and why.

How do you feel now about the most traumatic thing that has ever happened to you?

How did this trauma impact your life?

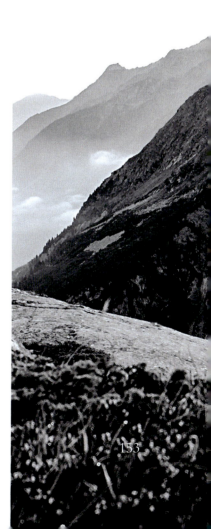

Time yourself for one minute. During the minute, write down as many words that begin with the letter "B" as you can.

How many did you write down?

If you wrote down 15 or more, good, your brain is working normally. If you only could write down 3-4 words that begin with the letter "B" you may be suffering from PTSD or Post-traumatic Stress Disorder. Alexander McFarlane found that people with PTSD struggled with focused attention and learning new information. This was one way he tested to find out if someone may be suffering from PTSD.

What was it like for that _____ year old to experience:

Write down what your _____ year old felt and thought about him or herself when this occurred in their life:

How do you feel about that little girl or boy who experienced:

Write down how you feel about him or her:

Can you allow that scared girl or boy to tell you what it had been like to:

Share how you felt when that happened to you as a little girl or boy:

EXTRA JOURNALING & DRAWING SPACE

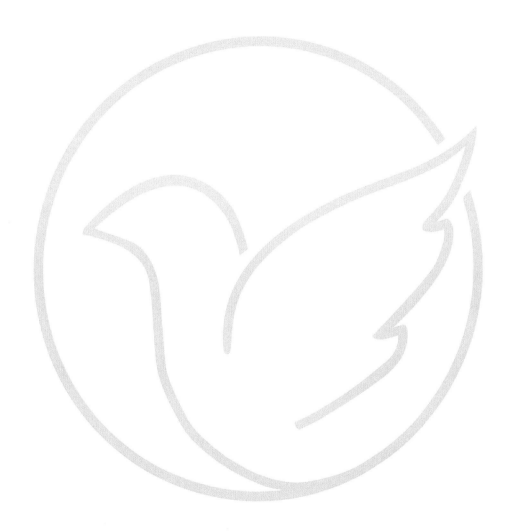

"An old belief is like an old shoe. We so value its comfort
that we fail to notice the hole in it."
~Robert Brault

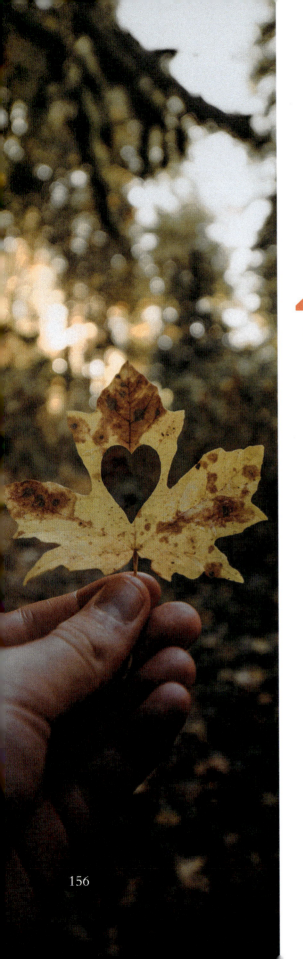

Section 3: Unraveling the Imprint of Trauma

Chapter 5

Healing The Abandoned Heart

What was the biggest thing that impacted you in this chapter and why?

"Nobody grows old merely by living a number of years. We grow old by deserting our ideals. Years may wrinkle the skin, but to give up enthusiasm wrinkles the soul."
~Samuel Ullman

"Statistically speaking, one-third to one-half of traumatized people will develop substance abuse problems. Drugs and alcohol provide temporary relief from trauma symptoms but as soon as drugs and alcohol are stopped, there is an increase in hyperarousal, nightmares, flashbacks and irritability."

Do you now or have you ever struggled with substance abuse problems? What type of addiction have you struggled with and why?

Do you use substances to avoid feelings from trauma, flashbacks or some of the lingering effects of trauma?

Are you ready to get help to stop substance abuse and resolve wounds from the past?

Have you ever gone to an AA meeting or a meeting to help with addiction problems?

If you want to work on an addiction problem, find a local AA meeting and work on the steps of AA.

AA's 12-Step approach follows a set of guidelines designed as "steps" toward recovery. Members can revisit these steps at any time. The 12 Steps are:

1. We admitted we were powerless over alcohol—that our lives had become unmanageable. Say out loud," My life has become unmanageable and I am powerless over my addiction."

2. We came to believe that a Power greater than ourselves could restore us to sanity. Say out loud, "I need help from God and a power greater than myself. God, help restore me to sanity. Give me the ability and the power to not rely on addictive substances to repress trauma and pain in my life."

3. Made a decision to turn our will and our lives over to the care of God, as we understood Him. Say out loud, "I decide to turn my will and life over to the care of God. God show me who you are. Help me to know you and rely upon you instead of addictive substances to manage my life. God, become real to me. I want a real relationship with you."

4. Made a searching and fearless moral inventory of ourselves. Write your moral inventory here. What do you do on a regular basis that you feel is wrong?
   _____
   _____
   _____
   _____

5. Admitted to God, ourselves and another human being the exact nature of our wrongs. Find a friend or talk to a pastor (they are not mandatory reporters like counselors) to admit what you have done that you feel is wrong. Ask God for forgiveness. Say out loud, "God, I'm sorry for _____. I know that it is wrong. I admit that I need help, I can't change myself and I am powerless over what I do wrong. Please help me and change me to be the person you want me to be."

6. Were entirely ready to have God remove all these defects of character. Say out loud, "God, I'm ready to have you remove all of the defects in my character. I can't fix myself and I see that I am powerless over certain behaviors in my life. I surrender my life to you and ask you to change me."

7. Humbly asked Him to remove our shortcomings. Say out loud, "Help me God and remove my shortcomings. I am imperfect and flawed, but you are perfect and can remove my flaws to make me right before your perfection."

8. Made a list of all persons we had harmed and became willing to make amends to them all. Write a list of those people you have wronged and what you need forgiveness for:

   1. Ask _____ for forgiveness for
   _____.

   2. Ask _____ for forgiveness for
   _____.

   3. Ask _____ for forgiveness for
   _____.

   4. Ask _____ for forgiveness for
   _____.

9. Made direct amends to such people wherever possible, except when to do so would injure them or others. Either write each person a letter to apologize and ask for forgiveness or take them out for coffee to apologize in person.

10. Continued to take personal inventory and when we were wrong promptly admitted it.

11. Sought through prayer and meditation to improve our conscious contact with God, as we understood Him, praying for knowledge of His will and the power to carry it out. Say out loud, "God help me to improve my conscious contact with you. Let me know the knowledge of your will for my life and empower me to live it out." Now, ask God a question and wait for an answer. "God, what is your will for my life?"

12. Having had a spiritual awakening as the result of these Steps, we tried to carry this message to alcoholics, and to practice these principles in all of our affairs. Say out loud, "God let me experience a spiritual awakening in my life that will change me and set me free from the need of addictive substances."

Alcoholics Anonymous World Services, Inc. (2016). The Twelve Steps of Alcoholics Anonymous.

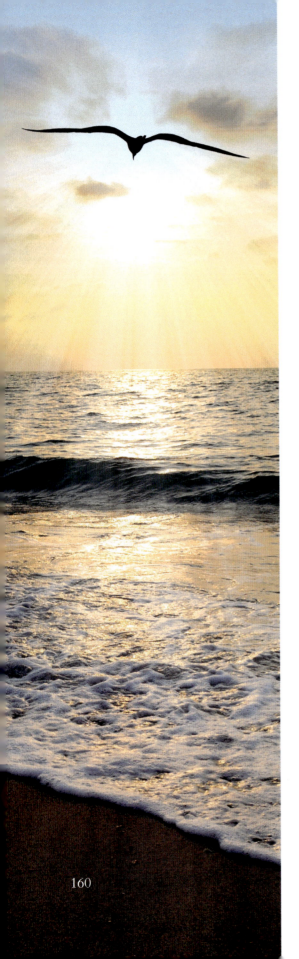

Section 4: Wakefulness

Chapter 1

Wake up to Spiritual Reality

What impacted you most in this chapter and why?

Has anyone in your life ever committed suicide or tried to commit suicide, including you?

How did their choice to commit suicide impact you?

Have you resolved the trauma involved in losing your loved one to suicide?

⎡ *If you have not been able to resolve the trauma of losing someone to suicide, seek professional help at the same time that you use the tools that we gave you in the chapter on memory work:* **Chapter 3: Freeing Your Mind From Imprints Of Trauma.** ⎤

What are the religious or spiritual backgrounds of you and your parents?

Have you had a positive experience with religion and/or spirituality or a negative experience and why?

What is your perspective on God?

Is God a friend, Father or distant authority figure?

How close do you feel to God? *If you don't know how to answer this, draw a picture to depict where you are in the world and where God is.*

What do you see in the picture that you drew? What does it mean?

Perform Logotherapy with yourself:

//

1. Have a project to work on every day, a reason to get out of bed in the morning and something that serves a need for others.

    What is the project that you can work on every day that gives you a powerful reason to get out of bed?

2. Have a redemptive perspective on life's challenges. When something traumatic happens in your life, find ways that you can pursue meaning or good to come out of suffering.

    What are the top 3 most traumatic things that have happened to you?

    _____
    _____
    _____

    Can you see anything good that came out of these situations? Write down 1 good thing that came out of each experience.

    _____
    _____
    _____

3. Share your life with a person or a community of people who love you unconditionally.

    Who is the person or community in your life currently who love you unconditionally?

    If you don't have this right now, how can you find this relationship or community?

Section 4: Wakefulness

Chapter 2

We all Have an Incurable Disease

What impacted you most in this chapter and why?

The spiritual realm is invisible, but the impact of the spiritual realm can be seen by the naked eye. The spiritual realm is mysterious and needs to be engaged in a particular way to find the connection that we seek. Let's look at the following categories of spiritual engagement to help you find your way to connect spiritually.

Purpose:

Finding our unique design or blueprint can offer a deep sense of spiritual fulfillment. The things that you are naturally inclined towards or naturally gifted in can be explored and developed towards this aim. What is your purpose on earth?

What are you naturally good at that other people notice about you as they get to know you?

Where do you find the most meaning and fulfillment in your life?

What do you do for other people that help them while giving you a sense of satisfaction at the same time?

When in your life have you felt the most like yourself? Why?

Intuition:

Some people learn to suppress their gut instinct out of a desire to please other people. Others learn to tune into their intuition and follow its guidance. Your gut instinct is usually about the future and what you need to do to navigate decision-making in the present.

When I was pregnant with my first son, Noble Thomas, I had a feeling that we should skip church one Sunday. I didn't know why, but I had a gut feeling that we should stay home.

Instead of listening to my intuition, we went to church. At the end of the service, we received an urgent phone call. My grandma was rushed to the hospital and was gravely ill. We hurried to the hospital to see her. She died the next morning.

We still got to see my grandma before she died. However, being pregnant at the time, I needed extra rest and consistent meals to feel balanced. My visit with my grandma was rushed because I needed to get home to rest and eat.

It would have been much better to stay at home because I would have been well-rested and not hungry when I was seeing my grandma for the last time. My spirit knew something about the future that I didn't know that day. Moments like that remind me to listen to my intuition and what it is telling me about the future.

Do you tend to listen to your gut feelings and make decisions based upon your intuition?

Do you ignore or steamroll over your intuition? Why or why not?

Do you remember times that you have ignored your intuition and suffered as a result? What happened?

Do you remember times that you have listened to your intuition and have been rewarded as a result?

Do an exercise this week. Every day for 7 days, make a point to tune into your intuition and decide to do what it is telling you to do instead of ignoring it. Record your results and what happens when you follow its guidance. What did you discover?

Death

The concept of death can be very challenging to navigate for people as it brings up a lot of fear when spiritual beliefs have not been solidified regarding death. It's important to work through your feelings while developing your beliefs surrounding death.

Let's explore this concept further to help you examine your beliefs about death or to help you find beliefs surrounding life after death. If you don't feel ready to die, if you don't feel peace-surrounding death or if you are facing a life-threatening illness like cancer and you want to prepare yourself for death, you may find this section invaluable.

How comfortable are you with the concept of death?

Do you feel ready to die? Why or why not?

Do you feel peace regarding death and what will happen after you die?
Why or why not?

Do you remember the first funeral that you went to when you were young?
How did you feel?

Was death explained to you by anyone when you were a child?
What did they say that you can remember now?

In general, when you go to a funeral, do you feel uncomfortable, fearful and sad about death? Why or why not?

Do you know anyone in your life that feels peaceful about death?

Have you ever asked them about their beliefs surrounding death and why they seem peaceful about dying? Now is your chance to ask them!

What do you believe happens after we die?

How confident are you that your beliefs are 100% accurate?

Do you feel that you have complicated grief as a result of not being free to grieve in a community setting?

How To Resolve Grief That Is Still Lingering:

Is there a retreat center near your home that offers bereavement retreats that you can schedule a weekend get away for you and other loved ones? My husband and I were given the gift of going to a bereavement center called Faith Lodge after the loss of our son. It helped tremendously in our grieving process.

Can you do a small memorial service with a few close friends or family members? For example, if you had a miscarriage and feel that you have not grieved the loss of your child, you can do a memorial service for closure. In the service, you can give your child a name and share your grief with those attending the service with you.

Every year, on Noble's birthday, we do a celebration for his birthday to remember him. Choose a day out of the year to remember and celebrate the person that you lost.

Plan a trip with a few close friends or family members to commemorate your loved one. Decide on activities and events that are meaningful. Spend some time reminiscing and sharing favorite memories about your loved one.

Create a scrapbook of your loved one. Involve friends and family members, asking for their best pictures. Write memories and notes in the scrapbook. When you are finished, throw a party and invite all who loved the person who is no longer with you. Share the scrapbook with everyone and a few words about your love and grief.

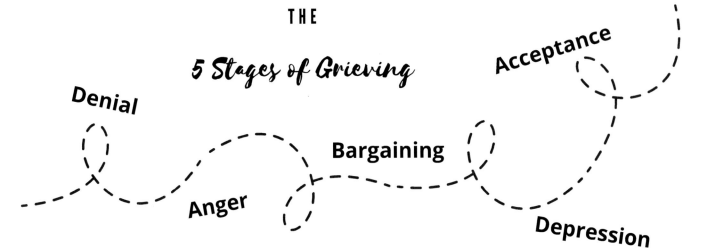

[It is easy to get stuck in a stage of grieving and not move past that particular stage. For example, some people choose to stay in the denial stage and avoid dealing with grief altogether.]

Think about the top 5 major losses in your life, where someone you loved died:

1.
2.
3.
4.
5.

Imagine each loss and discover if you made it to the acceptance stage. Focus on the image of the person you lost and attempt to discover how you feel.

Do you feel numb?
Do you feel angry?
Do you feel depressed?
Do you have any unresolved grief in your life?

Do you feel confused?
Do you feel peace and acceptance?

What do you plan on doing to engage in the grieving process again to fully accept the loss?

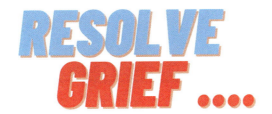

Consider this excerpt from the book:

"In his research, David Spiegel found that being able to express emotions like anger and grief can improve survival rates in cancer. I often think about what it would feel like to still carry the trauma, emotional pain and weight of the loss of Noble in my body."

Can you express emotions like anger and grief well or do you struggle with this? Why or why not?

Do you still carry grief and trauma in your body?

Where is it located in your body?

Why is it still there?

What is one good thing about aging that can help you embrace aging as a concept?

In light of what you learned about regarding the nocebo effect & cancer, do you think it is ethical for oncologists to give a time frame of how long someone has to live?

Has your oncologist given you a time frame on how long they expect you to be alive?

1. How did you feel after you were given this time frame?

2. Are you feeding into The Nocebo Effect instead of The Placebo Effect as a result?

3. Did it cause you to lose hope and give up on your healing?

4. Say the following prayer with me, **"God, I forgive my doctor,_____, for telling me that I have only ____ months or years to live. I reject their conclusion on the matter. Instead, I submit my life to you and trust that you can extend my life."**

EXTRA JOURNALING & DRAWING SPACE

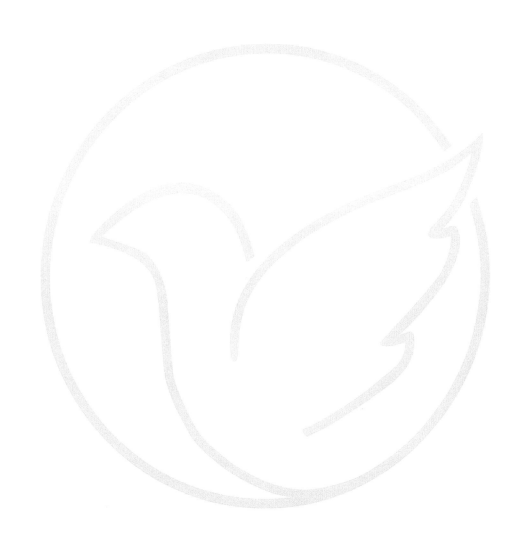

"The measure of a life, after all, is not its duration, but its donation."
~*Corrie Ten Boom*

Meditation surrounding finding peace regarding death:

I want to lead you in a meditation to help you find peace surrounding death if you do not already have peace surrounding the concept of death.

Close your eyes. As you close your eyes, allow yourself to feel all of the feelings you have surrounding death. Remember times that you went to funerals of loved ones to help access your feelings surrounding death. Draw a picture about how you feel about death:

What do you notice about this picture?

_____
_____
_____
_____
_____

Now, close your eyes again. Surrender control and invite God to communicate with you. I want you to ask God a few questions, wait and listen for the answers. **Remember, we are not trying to listen to our own beliefs.** We are trying to access answers from God to get a different perspective than we carry currently:

Why am I afraid of death?

How do I find peace surrounding death?

How do you feel about death?

What happens after we die?

How do I make peace with death?

> **Questions about Worldview:**
> Spirituality is defined as we allow ourselves to ask tough questions and seek out the answers. Every night before I went to bed when I was 5-12 years old, I would have questions about spirituality run through my head.

I never asked them out loud, but I was very curious and had basic questions that lingered in my mind. The questions that I had as a child were:

1. *Where did I come from?*
2. *Who is God?*
3. *Why am I here?*
4. *Where did the earth come from?*

Did you also have questions like this as a child?

Were your questions answered or were they left unanswered?

Let's go through some worldview questions to see where you are at with your worldview. If you still have some holes in your worldview, you may want to follow the questions to find the answers that you seek.

Worldview meditation:

Open your mind & close your eyes. Try to let go of any expectations or any preconceived ideas about the spiritual world. Be open to a surprise. Ask questions & wait for the answers to come to you from the spiritual realm, not from yourself:

- Who is God?

- Is there a God?

- What is truth?

- Is there absolute truth?

- What is love?

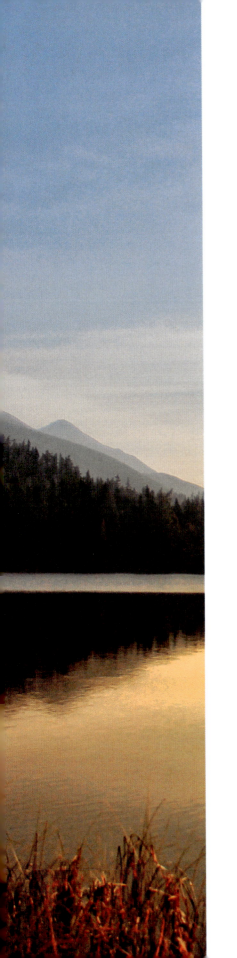

- What is morality? Who defines morality?

- Where did life originate?

- What happens when we die?

- What is the purpose of life?

- Do I have the ability to make free choices?

Dreams:

Dreams are the spiritual realm's way of communicating to us.
I have had dreams that have given me direction in life and critical revelation about myself. I have had dreams that have literally healed me and transformed my desires. In addition, I have had dreams that have told me about the future to give me hope in a hard season.

Do you remember your dreams?

Are they vivid and clear in their meaning to you?

Have you had a vivid dream that spoke to you deeply or changed your life?

What was it?

Are you open to dream and receive messages from the spiritual realm or are you spiritually closed?

Do an exercise with me. Buy a journal specifically intended to be a dream journal. Set the dream journal by your bed with a pen. Say the following out loud, **"God I am open for you to communicate to me through dreams. I want to receive understanding and revelation through my dreams. Speak to me through my dreams and help me to understand their meaning. Remove anything that would block me from receiving dreams from you."**

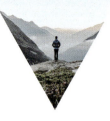

Conscience

Your conscience imprints on your psychology what is right and wrong and what you should or should not do. Sometimes we rebel against our conscience and our sense of right and wrong and sometimes we align ourselves with our conscience to do what we think is right in a given situation.

○─────────────────────────○

Your conscience is different than your intuition as your conscience comes from your mind instead of your gut. Your conscience is a generalized sense of right or wrong and not based upon decision-making for the future.

> Do you tend to listen to and obey your conscience or are you in a habit of rebelling against the instructions that your conscience gives you?

_____
_____
_____
_____

Take this next week to tune into your conscience.
What is it telling you? What is it telling you to do that is right and what is it telling you to avoid?

Resolving regrets:

Close your eyes and picture the event where you broke your own moral law. If you hurt someone, in the memory, ask for forgiveness.

**Please forgive me, _____,
for_____. I am sorry for hurting you.**

Wait and receive forgiveness.
If you are open to it, also ask God to forgive you for your moral transgression.

**God, I am sorry for _____.
I broke my own sense of right and wrong when I did that and I hurt you, others and myself. Please remove the pain of this regret.**

Do this exercise for every regret you can think of in your past.

Now, take a moment to recommit to live according to your moral compass and ask God to help you. Say the following out loud, **"God, help me to live according to my moral compass and to do what is right. Forgive me for where I have messed up and done what is wrong morally."**

....
....
....
....

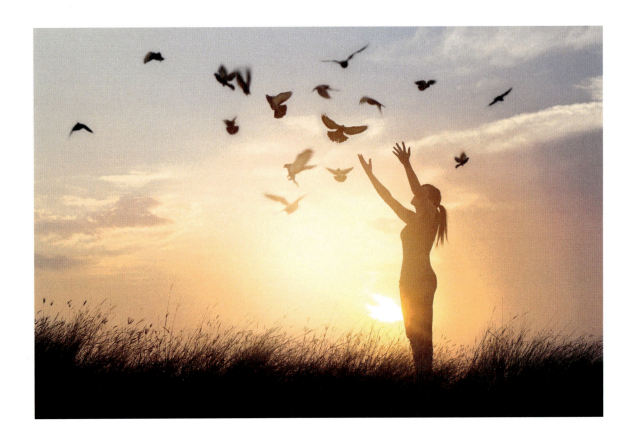

Peace:

Some people have a generalized sense of anxiety because of the lack of spiritual pursuit and spiritual development. If you are at that place where you are anxious and need peace, just ask for peace.

Say out loud, **"God, I ask you to help me. I am struggling with a lot of anxiety and I don't know why. Can you give me peace?"**

Now wait to receive the peace that the spiritual realm has to give you.

Jesus:

People and religions have differing opinions about Jesus. Some say that he was a prophet, others say he was a teacher and a moral man, others claim that he was God in the flesh. In the end, only what you believe about Jesus matters. Let's explore your beliefs.

What were your beliefs about Jesus growing up? Do you believe that they are true or untrue?

Have you ever asked God who Jesus is?
Say the following out loud, **"God, I'm unsure what to believe regarding Jesus. I ask you humbly and openly, who is Jesus?"**
Now, wait for God to reply. What do you hear or see?

Did you receive the gift of righteousness from Jesus at the end of the book, *Braving The Storm*? What happened when you did?

For those who did receive the gift of righteousness from Jesus and you want to take it one step further, say this prayer with me, **"Thank you God for the life of Jesus. I believe in my heart and confess with my mouth that Jesus is Lord. Thank you for forgiving me. I receive the gift of the Holy Spirit now. Empower me to live for you and to know you in a personal way. Show me the reality of Jesus. Amen."**

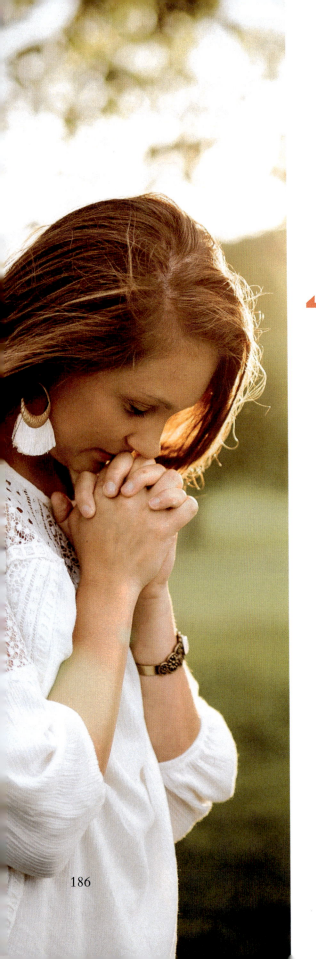

Conclusion

"The end of a matter is better then its beginning."
~Ancient Proverb

We pray and hope that you have experienced a profound, internal transformation after reading the book, *Braving The Storm*, and following the exercises in this companion workbook.

Now, you are ready for the final assessment.

- Why did you have cancer?

- What are 3 new things that you are aware of about yourself after this book and workbook?

- Why did you develop cancer:
    - Relationally?

    - Emotionally?

    - Physically?

    - Spiritually?

Have you increased or improved your spiritual connection? How?

In what ways did you allow areas of your life to die prior to a cancer diagnosis and how have you come alive again?

What was the biggest revelation that you gained in reading this book and doing the workbook?

What have you been able to resolve from your past as you have read *Braving The Storm* and gone through this workbook?

What was your profound, internal transformation?

EXTRA JOURNALING & DRAWING SPACE

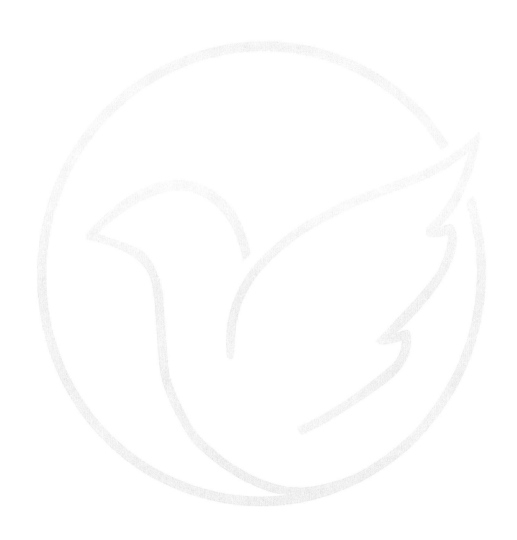

"We look forward to the time when the power of love will replace the love of power. Then will our world know the blessings of peace."
~*William Ewart Gladstone*

STOP BY
www.cancerpeaceuniversity.com

SHOP
www.cancerpeaceuniversity.com

SEND A NOTE
cancerpeaceuniversity@gmail.com

CONNECT
Cancer Peace University

If you want to share your story with us, email us at **cancerpeaceuniversity@gmail.com** and we will be excited to hear your amazing story!

Cancer Peace University trains all holistic practitioners, doctors and nutritional therapists who have a fear of working with cancer patients or who are passionate about helping their clients promote longevity. Our goal is to guide clients to promote longevity, to train the next generation of holistic practitioners to work with those diagnosed with cancer and to fund orphanage work.

Month Day Year
END DATE

Made in the USA
Las Vegas, NV
26 June 2023

73919845R00117